RECOVERED

How I transformed my life from miserable to miraculous & how you can too

Judy Morris

RECOVERED: How I transformed my life from miserable to miraculous & how you can too, is a work of my own creation.

This book does not replace the advice of a medical professional or trained therapist. Consult your physician or mental health professional before making any changes to your health plan.

To maintain the anonymity of any individuals involved in situations detailed within, I have changed some names, details, and specific telling characteristics.

The information in this book was correct at the time of publication, and the Author does not assume any liability for loss or damage caused by errors or omissions, again, this is my perspective, opinion, and experience, so it has been written as such.

ISBN 979-8-9865393-8-6 (paperback)
ISBN 979-8-9865393-7-9 (ebook)

Author Photo by Libby Danforth
Cover, Book Design, and Layout by megs thompson, megswrites llc

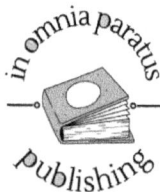

in omnia paratus publishing

www.inomniaparatuspublishing.com

Advance Praise

"Just finished this brilliant book. One of many continued contributions for the silent sufferers and seasoned survivors. So much resonance throughout. Much like other study guides, this will be a reference more than just a read that only gets a once over than ends up on a shelf. There's so much insight and guidance that beckons revisiting specific sentences for one's own prolonged pondering and review."

Renee Kische, Real Estate Investor

"RECOVERED is the perfect combination of personal accountability and understanding the way that trauma/ family dynamics impact us. A quote from the book that stood out to me the most is "we cannot meet anyone on a deeper level than we have met ourselves!" So important and powerful. I also appreciated the discussion about western culture and the way that we relate our worth to our accomplishments - it was so impactful.

Thank you for illuminating the importance of taking accountability in our lives, having a team, and untethering ourselves from sick family dynamics/ cultural messages. I appreciated the way that you discussed actions that people can take on multiple levels (and despite disabilities etc.), I think that it empowers people to make a change regardless of their financial resources or capabilities. I think that the message is super inclusive, and people could relate it to anything that they are struggling with. I am so blessed to have such an incredible coach to guide me in creating a miraculous life!"

Ashley Morrison, Counselor

"RECOVERED is astoundingly beautiful, profound, and deeply impactful. Thank you for writing about PTSD and Trauma in such an

accessible and succinct way. Furthermore, each sentence and paragraph are well written with precision and interlaced with deep knowledge about each of the issues and associated healing modalities. Beyond the healings, I appreciated your vulnerability in telling your story in such a deep and intensely candid way. I am grateful to have you as a coach and guide to help me create miracles in my life."

Summer Swigart, Tech Executive

"RECOVERED is a beautifully written book about an unbeautiful subject matter. Judy shared her story with candor, courage, and vulnerability. Sharing insights and knowledge in a way that was clear and easy to understand. I couldn't put it down, it was riveting."

Bill MacDonald, Retired Tech Executive

To every person who ever felt alone or afraid, helpless, or ashamed. I know how it is and how you wish it could be. It will get better IF you are willing to do the work.

Table of Contents

Disclaimer

Please be advised that this book deals with sensitive issues such as substance abuse, alcoholism, codependency, love addiction, depression, PTSD, and other mental health issues. This book expresses controversial views on society, familial, and current cultural patterns. It was written with the intent to disrupt the existing paradigms, encouraging you to question your existing views of yourself, your beliefs, and your challenges. However, it was not written to provide any kind of diagnosis or advice.

The author is not a licensed therapist or medical practitioner of any kind. She is simply a person sharing her experience and personal journey of recovery. Please do not construe any of the information provided in this book as advice. Be sure to consult a licensed medical professional before making any decisions regarding your mental health.

Judy Morris

My Story: What's Wrong with Me?!

What's wrong with me? This is the question I was born with. As a small child, I couldn't help but feel that there was something wrong with me. There was inherent anxiety in the background of my being - feeling insecure, unsteady, and unsure about who I was and what my place was in the world.

I was born in a small town in East Los Angeles to a single mother of 23. My parents separated before I was born. My mother was young, alone, and had to work multiple positions to support the two of us. Luckily my grandparents were available to help, and they played a critical role in my upbringing. I never met my biological father. I never had the opportunity to ask him why it was, he wasn't a part of my life, and while I may never know his reason, I can only imagine that he truly didn't know or believe that I was his. I see this as being the only reason he may have been justified in dropping out of the equation. I cannot imagine that his absence from my life was intended to cause damage.

My mother's lack of insistence that he submitted to a paternity test to corroborate her allegations was not intended to harm me either. My mother was not guilty of malice, but naivety and pride. Given her lack of emotional maturity and psychological education, she had no way of knowing how his absence would impact my life and my identity. I had no idea as a small child that the absence of those things would create a core wound of abandonment, leaving me depressed and vulnerable. As I reached adolescence, alcoholism and co-dependency would become the cure for that.

There is no cookie-cutter recipe for success or disaster when raising a child as we each react differently to challenging circumstances and some

3

children fare better than others. There is no way to measure inherent resilience in a child that can only be measured as it is witnessed in their development over the course of a lifetime.

Although children are technically born blank slates barring severe circumstances (severe illness with the mother, birth defects, etc.) they do not arrive here with insecurities and neurosis. Such maladies manifest in conjunction with their genetic imprint, the circumstances by which they are brought into the world, how they are brought into the world, and how they are nurtured. Over the last decade, there has been extensive research that has expanded the literature on epigenetics and inherited trauma, clinicians and scientists have been investigating the ways in which trauma is transmitted from one generation to the next, how it's held in our minds and bodies, and expressed as our own. Studies have shown that our ancestor's trauma is passed down as what celebrated psychoanalyst Galit Atlas calls an emotional inheritance, leaving a trace in our minds and in those of future generations.

Galit states: "in the end, we come to realize that it is the unexamined lives of our parents that we ourselves end up living." Therefore, the greatest gift a child can receive is a caregiver who has already begun the work of unpacking their family's emotional inheritance and healing their own nervous systems so that they can provide their children with an environment suitable for developing intact nervous systems and secure attachments. Secure attachments begin with caregivers who are present, and self-regulated, who create emotional, physical safety, support, and structure for a child's development. When children know that they are protected and are not concerned about their basic needs being met, providing them with a deep sense of belonging to their family and community, they are able to relax and just be. Their personalities can develop organically vs. becoming parentified and catapulted into premature adulthood as a trauma response to unfavorable circumstances. When children are born into insecure circumstances, with caregivers who lack maturity, emotional intelligence, education, and self-awareness, as well as extreme poverty, they are prone to suffer a variety of consequences such as mental health issues manifesting as anxiety, depression, hyperactivity, or behavioral problems acted out in the home, academic, and social lives. It may, later, manifest in physical health problems such as reduced immunity, asthma, and heart disease to name a few.[1]

I was impacted greatly by not having a traditional family structure to rely on, especially growing up and spending much of my formative years with my grandparents who belonged to a church where the central theme was based not only on basic Christian doctrine but with a rigorous focus around the importance of a traditional nuclear family.

Every Sunday I would attend church, surrounded by my peers, their siblings, and their parents. We sang songs about families. FAMILY. FAMILY. FAMILY. It was as if my desire to be a part of a loving family was being thrown in my face. I felt powerless in the knowledge that I didn't have a traditional family, and deep down I felt ashamed of my existence. I knew I was a bastard. I knew I wasn't born into the bonds of holy matrimony. Given everything I was learning at church and how different it was from what I was living at home, I felt more and more insecure and ashamed of my existence. Of course, at the time I had no awareness of this. I just knew that I felt miserable and depressed, and I had no idea why.

---

[1] For additional information watch Dr. Nadine Burk Harris' TEDTalk @ https://www.ted.com/talks/nadine_burke_harris_how_childhood_trauma_aff ects_health_across_a_lifetime

Judy Morris

I adored my grandfather who was my best friend and subsequent Higher Power. As far as I was concerned the sun rose and set in his eyes. However, loving him wasn't easy. He had severe depression, anxiety, and was struggling with his own mental health. My grandmother was struggling with her own diminished physical health and the imposed limitations of her illnesses. As much as they loved me, they didn't have the emotional or financial resources to raise a child, facts I was painfully aware of. It left me feeling like an imposition on their lives. I hated feeling like a burden and soon began a lifelong quest to become the most independent, resourceful person possible. My goal in life was to never need anyone.

As imperfect of a scenario as it was, I was content to be with my grandparents. As much as my mother adored me and wanted to provide a stable home life, she could not. She was busy working full time in addition to managing a successful career in entertainment, where she was a highly sought-after performer, while simultaneously trying to manage a tumultuous love life in addition to struggling with a variety of her own health issues.

I thought for sure that everything was going to be ok and then BAM. Just like that, everything changed. My grandparents decided they were going to sell their home and move to the Pacific Northwest. That in and of itself wasn't the issue for me. The issue was that they were not going to take me with them. My fragile self-esteem was on thin ice to begin with, and my already shaky sense of stability was gone in a flash. I was left to live with my mother who at the time was in the midst of the most abusive, unstable relationship of her life. I was in a crisis and there was no one coming to my rescue. Just like that, any faith I had in a Higher Power vanished. My faith in my grandparents vanished. My will to live vanished. It was the most suicidally depressed experience of my life, and I was only 12 years old.

To make matters worse no one acknowledged my plight. The loss and grief I experienced were devastating. I was barely functioning and being told to stop being so dramatic, to pull myself together. My feelings had never been so invalidated. I had no one to turn to, save for my beloved school counselor who did her utmost to provide me with compassion and understanding but even that wasn't sufficient. It wasn't until that summer when I discovered Marlboro Red's and Miller High Life that things changed for me.

I hadn't grown up in a home with alcohol. Certainly, alcoholism was in the background of our lives, as my mother had a habit of falling in love with men who were afflicted, but she never allowed them to drink in our home so although I was exposed to untreated alcoholism and codependency, I was not exposed to the act of drinking itself. So, it never occurred to me that drinking could be a solution, until one fateful summer afternoon when I skipped my summer school classes.

Out on the lawn adjacent to the high school where I was taking classes, I sat in a circle with a group of teens a few years older than myself. They were passing around a red plastic party cup filled with a mixture of Boones Strawberry Hill and Thunderbird. I had already developed a habit of smoking, but before that day, I'd never taken a drink. The cup made its way around the circle, everyone taking a sip before passing it along. When the red cup reached me, I thought to myself, it's no big deal, it's just alcohol. With that first drink, it was love at first sip. From the moment it hit my lips, stung my throat, and warned my lungs it felt as though a cozy blanket had been wrapped around me. Suddenly all the angst that was a constant in the background of my existence dissipated and I could breathe. My love affair with drinking and subsequent alcoholism was born at that moment. At first, everything was great. It was the solution that helped me cope with the feelings that were too big to feel, the circumstances that were outside my control. It was a magical cure-all that provided comfort, pleasure, and confidence in an instant.

My mother was not happy about my discovery. She was diligent about not allowing any of her partners to drink in our home, and she was no less militant when it came to me. Of course, that didn't stop me. I continued drinking. She continued to catch me, and I suffered the consequences of my actions, but it was no matter. I would have paid any price for that sense of peace. Ultimately my home life became untenable as my mother, and I had irreconcilable differences. The insanity of the relationship she had with the man in her life escalated and I knew deep in my heart that it was time for me to go. As difficult as this realization was for my mother, I can never express my gratitude to her for understanding this fact and for her generosity in making the necessary arrangements for me to have another place to live. That remains the most loving and selfless act she ever performed on my behalf.

She connected me with an older couple in our neighborhood who were very happy to have me in their home. It was the perfect combination of freedom and structure. They were the best people in the whole world as far as I was concerned and that was one of the happiest periods of my life. I was finally at peace which enabled me to finish High School successfully.

The first 4 years of my drinking were golden. Alcohol worked beautifully and was my foolproof solution. I was happy because for the first time, I was experiencing a sense of ease and comfort that had alluded me throughout my life until that point.

All of that changed after high school. As wonderful as things were in my new home, my boyfriend at the time wanted us to get a place of our own. It seemed logical, like the next step in life so I agreed. Looking back, I can see now how this move was not what I wanted, but at that time in my life, I didn't have enough self-esteem, self-awareness, or courage to ask for what I actually wanted. All I knew was survival and maintaining the relationship with my boyfriend was a survival tactic, although I couldn't have recognized it as such at the time.

I had no idea what was coming. It never dawned on me that until that point, I'd been able to "control" my drinking, if for no reason other than because I had to keep up appearances for others and wasn't able to drink excessively while living with that older couple. That changed, once I was in a home of my own with no supervision, there was no need to control myself, and my drinking skyrocketed.

Judy Morris

What Went Wrong?

Some people can drink lots and lots of alcohol daily, but I could not. It was wreaking havoc on my physical and mental health. The decline in both had been so rapid that within a few short months I crashed into a pitiful and incomprehensible demoralization and recognized that I needed help, so I decided to attend a 12-step meeting.

I remember like it was yesterday. I had 72 hours sober, and I was unsteady, tearful, and uncertain about the future. Who was I? Where was the confident, carefree girl who fancied herself independent, sophisticated, and unaffected by anyone or anything? She had disappeared into a bottle and couldn't find her way out. I was a bundle of nerves, shaking like a leaf. I realize now that my condition had simply been the result of me stuffing my feelings, avoiding my fears, and ignoring my trauma. I had been depressed all my life, pretending I wasn't, and alcohol had been the perfect prop, helping me perpetuate my own illusion that everything was ok. Until it wasn't. When my servant became my master, and everything turned on me I was finally faced with my feelings, and they were so overwhelming I couldn't be with them. At first, I thought that I just had a drinking problem and that if I stopped drinking everything would be ok. I didn't know that once I stopped drinking, I would FEEL better. I would feel pain better, fear better, anxiety better, insecurity better. I would FEEL everything.

I didn't know that there had been so much pain to mask. I didn't know that I was suffering from anything. I thought that I enjoyed drinking and that it was fun and social. I hadn't thought about it any further than that.

Deep down, I knew that the trauma that had occurred when I was 12 years old had been a terrible experience but what I didn't know was that I

11

had buried all the feelings associated with that trauma which only compounded the feelings and traumas that came before that. All my experiences, memories, fears, and insecurities were still there like an infection waiting to escalate and take me down.

Sobriety didn't feel empowering, healthy, or positive. It felt terrifying, catastrophic, and unsustainable. I found myself in a mental health crisis that I could never have anticipated. The first 30 days of my sobriety were tough. I had panic attacks so severe that I ended up in my doctor's office, being prescribed antidepressants. They didn't help, not really. There wasn't anything that could help. I was in a pain so deep and so profound that nothing seemed to suppress it. Not even alcohol could help anymore. I stopped drinking because it stopped working. I didn't know where to go from there.

I came to the realization that I needed to stay sober, and to stay sober I had to break up with my boyfriend and move out. Perhaps that doesn't sound like a big deal for a young girl to break up with her boyfriend - but for me, it wasn't so simple.

I didn't have close ties with my family, and I was very close to his. My identity was wrapped up in my relationship with him, and the sense of safety and comfort I felt by being in that relationship. I found myself struck with the realization that if I stayed with him, I would not be able to stay sober and I knew that I had to stay sober at all costs. As terrifying as it was to leave him and our life together, I knew that there was nothing left for me there. I knew that if I stayed, I wouldn't just be choosing him, I would be choosing to remain the same, to continue to drink and I couldn't do that to myself. I knew that there was no other choice. So, I did one of the bravest things I had ever done - I left.

Gratefully, a dear friend of mine had a room coming available in her three-bedroom apartment and until then, she allowed me to sleep on her couch. I was only 18 years old. I was so young and so alone but so determined to stay sober. I went to meetings and bought a big book, but I didn't open it and I didn't have a sponsor. I was on dangerous ground, and I didn't even know it.

Slowly my days turned into weeks and my weeks into months, the antidepressants started working and my panic attacks subsided. I was working and maintaining a cute little home with my friend and life was good - until it wasn't.

I met him. And that was that.

I didn't realize it then, but underneath it all, my alcoholism, depression, anxiety, and fear, I believed that the answer to all my problems lie in finding a man who would love me like no man had loved me before. Someone who would be there for me like no one had been there for me, who would make up for all the things that I didn't have growing up, like a father. It was a tall order I know, but I truly believed "he" existed and that "he" was the answer. I had the story memorized. We would fall madly in love, complete each other like in the movies, and ride off into the sunset together.

Given that I hadn't done any work on myself, the stability that I had created was short-lived. You see, I hadn't changed. I hadn't healed. All I had done was stop drinking and attend a few 12-step meetings. I had merely postponed the work that would inevitably need to be done to transform my life. I had yet to discover that it had never been my circumstances causing me pain, but my relationship with myself. I continued to create painful circumstances that perpetuated painful patterns. There was so much that I didn't know.

As stated above, I met that man and projected all my expectations and fantasies onto him, and he did the same to me in his own way. We became each other's prisoners trapped in a co-dependent, love-addicted cycle that was fraught with jealousy, accusations, and fighting.

As painful as it was, I was totally addicted to it. I was addicted because it made me feel important. No one had ever paid that much attention to me, tracked my every move. In some ways, it was like being a celebrity. I had no peace, I had to account for every moment. Being his possession felt like belonging and I ached to belong. My life became about obedience, and my mission was to become whoever he wanted me to be.

He didn't like me saying I was an alcoholic, so I stopped saying it. He didn't like me going to "those meetings" so I stopped going. He said I didn't need to take medication, so I stopped taking my antidepressants. I promoted him to the status of my Higher Power, and he happily accepted. My world became very small and after 2.5 years of living in that small world, I drank again.

If my man had had any doubts about my alcoholism before, I'm confident that after he saw who I became when I drank, all doubt was removed. I became a completely different person than the woman he had been living with. The insanity between us escalated and he became increasingly violent. I knew that if I didn't leave, I wouldn't survive. I truly believed he was capable of anything and there was still some small part of me that wanted to live.

Through all this turmoil, I had started a career in financial services and had some very exciting and promising things ahead of me. I turned my focus from romance to finance and switched obsessions from relationships to career. I got a transfer from one branch of my firm to another and rented a room from a friend. I did my utmost to move on. It took three full years of going back and forth on and off, in this toxic relationship before it had fully ended.

I firmly believe - because it has been my experience, that if nothing changes, nothing changes. Drinking was but a symptom, and although it was a problem it was not THE problem. It is not enough just to stop drinking. Alcoholism doesn't reside in a bottle; it resides in my mind, in my behavior. It resides inside of a wounded character who's developed a warped perception of themselves and the world.

All the unhealed wounds, resentments, regrets, unfulfilled expectations, betrayals, broken heartedness, and unfulfilled dreams find a dark corner of the mind in which to hide. One that resembles a cave. Sobriety is only a beginning. Yes, one must become physically sober to start, but if we are to truly heal, we must grow, and growth demands change. To move forward, I had to go back to that cave and begin excavation. I needed to examine under the light of the 12-steps with the guidance of a sponsor, therapist, psychiatrist, etc. all my troubles.

I had to get down to causes and conditions. Until I admitted and accepted my devastating weakness and all their consequences, my recovery would continue to be on shaky ground. I had relapsed in my relationship because I had gone from depending on alcohol to depending on a man/relationship (*switching addictions*) and since I hadn't done any work on myself, I ended up right back where I started, but this time it was worse because I was involved with someone violent and emotionally unstable.

In January 2002 I began my healing journey but this time with integrity, and commitment. I was completely invested in myself and my recovery. It had taken me 7 years and multiple attempts before I finally surrendered.

I had always known deep down inside that I needed help and that the way I had been doing things simply didn't work because I always ended up drunk and miserable. But I was too afraid to ask for help. I was full of fear and pride. Instead, I tried every which way to turn my life around on my own and it simply wasn't possible, I couldn't do it alone. I finally accepted that fact. After all, the first word in the first step is WE.

One of the biggest challenges I discovered as I faced my addiction was wanting there to be a third option. If you are a real alcoholic like I am, there are only two options: 1) go on drinking to ultimate destruction or 2) complete abstinence supported by a life of recovery. There is no option number three.

I had spent 7 years in and out of 12-step meetings trying a million different ways to find that elusive third option only to realize that it didn't exist. My choices were to continue living the way I had been, destroying myself and my life, or I could stop drinking for good, and learn a new way to live. Those were my options and at last, I surrendered. Finally, I was willing, and I took the leap.

I wish I could tell you where that willingness came from, how I got there. I think it's a combination of radical self-honesty, humility, and a desire to thrive, combined with a willingness to go to any length necessary, to not go back to the bottle.

I am deeply grateful that I finally heard the message and embraced it with my whole heart. In reality, I had no idea what I was stepping into. I had no clue what it would really take. The only thing I would have to change was everything. But I was ready, whatever recovery would ask of me, I would give. I was finally willing and ready.

I had spent my life giving myself away to people who really didn't care about me. Chasing men, relationships, and career success. Looking for something on the outside to make me feel ok on the inside.

Finally, I gave myself away to something worthy of me, by giving myself fully to my recovery. I committed to learning how to give to myself. I committed to learning how to repair my relationship with myself and how to develop a relationship with a real Higher Power, not the man-made Higher Power otherwise known as the holy trinity of western civilization: POWER, PROPERTY, and PRESTIGE wrapped up in a tidy package of self-obsession, the pursuit of phony Hollywood romance, and materialism.

I got busy. I got a sponsor, I went to a meeting every day, and I got a therapist. I knew I needed to figure out what the causes and conditions were of my self-destructive behavior and my depression, so I went to work on myself.

I discovered that all my failures, chronic disappointment, and lack of fulfillment were a result of ignorance. I had built a character on a foundation of fear fueled by ego. I was totally ignorant to who I was, how the Universe operated, and how life worked in general.

I had been operating from fear — fear of being worthless, unlovable, and alone covered up with the grandiosity of arrogance and lone rangerism. I had believed at my core that I didn't need anyone. I was dishonorable in my relationships with men, manipulating them for affection, attention, and "love." I was consumed with work-a-holism, working around the clock, trying to maintain the façade of being "wonder woman" chasing accomplishments yet feeling more and more empty at the end of the day.

Through the healing process, I became whole and complete for myself. I stopped surviving and started living. I learned how to dream again, how to value myself and others. I gained access to my creativity. I re-discovered the magic of connection and collaboration.

I discovered that real success could not be found in my bank account or relationship status. That success was about wholeness, balance, and contribution. I learned that if I got connected to my divine identity and lived by spiritual principles on a foundation of integrity instead of living my life based on the whims of my feelings and opinions, that I could live a miraculous life. And I have done just that. I am so excited to share my story, my journey with you. This is why I've written this book, to take all that I've learned over the last 20 years in my own recovery and break it down into a simple, easy-to-understand, and easy-to-use concept and design for living that can enable anyone, to live their own miraculous life.

It All Depends on You

As Doris Day crooned in the memorable 1955 film, "Love Me or Leave Me," "it all depends on you." And for so many of us that live or have previously lived in the land of codependency, how I feel about me truly does depend on you.

In western culture, we tend to deify the family structure. We deify our mothers, our fathers, and the very concept of family. How we feel about ourselves is largely connected to how our families feel about us. I cannot tell you how many clients I've worked with that think of themselves as incapable after a lifetime of their parent or guardian telling them so.

Deification is dangerous. It puts the object on a pedestal, out of reach — it's a construct devoid of humanity that objectifies all parties putting one above the other, leaving those beneath it in servitude to an ideal, value, concept, or person/group.

If I have idealized the concept or the values of my family, it impedes my ability to see them clearly and if I cannot see them clearly then I cannot see myself clearly. It's impossible to stand eye to eye with someone above me.

It's important to understand the truth of my identity. I come from divine spirit. I come through my parents, not from them.

The cosmic law that states like begets like means that it's impossible for an apple tree to produce pears or for a horse to give birth to a cat. Offspring must be of the same nature as the parent and so since God is divine spirit, man must essentially be divine spirit as well.

It's so important to understand our own divine identities, as well as the connection we have to our Higher Power. If we've mistakenly promoted our family or parents to that position, it interferes with the relationship we

19

form with our one true Source, or Higher Power. It's critical that we distinguish the difference between our relationships with our family and our relationships with our Source. Our freedom, prosperity, and abundance depend upon it.

It's quite natural for a small child to look up into the face of their mother or father and see a God-like image. Children only know their parents and don't yet possess a knowledge of who their Higher Power is, instead, by nature, they look to their parent or guardian to provide for their every need. As we mature, the process of individuation includes coming to terms with the truth of the nature of being, that our parents are human. They are not gods. And although we can love and respect them, if we place too much emphasis on their status, perfection, or importance - it dehumanizes them and interferes with our relationship with Source.

Our families are where we learn how to love and how to live. If in our most formative years we've experienced love being abusive, dysfunctional, or unhealthy, we're unable to recognize that this is wrong, because it's what we've always known, the way it's always been, and we'll continue to honor those traditions and values, passing them down to our own children, continuing a line of dysfunction.

There are so many sides to this story. This doesn't only refer to blatant dysfunction such as violence or substance abuse. There are many instances where children grow up in seemingly functional families. For example, if a child's parents own a thriving business, the natural expectation may be placed upon the children to perform academically, preparing themselves to one day take on the family business.

This may sound wonderful at first, but what if the child has different aspirations? What if the child doesn't want to go into the family business and wants to pursue something different like a career as a writer or an entertainer?

I've seen time and time again individuals squashed and suffocated living inside of rules that were assigned to them through their family. Seemingly prosperous and positive roles, but roles that robbed them of their creativity, authenticity, and self-expression.

If we are obligated and beholden to fulfill the expectations of our family than we are in a cage and no matter how plush or gilded that cage may be, a cage is still a cage.

In the United States, the Trafficking Victims Protection Act of 2000 (TVPA) defines labor trafficking as: "The recruitment, harboring, transportation, provision, or obtaining of a person for labor or services, through the use of force, fraud, or coercion for the purpose of subjection to involuntary servitude, peonage, debt bondage, or slavery" (22 USC § 7102(9)). See the Federal Laws page for more detailed definitions.

I cannot tell you how many adult children I've worked with that are being managed by their families as assets and therefore enslaved. They're being forced through coercion and threat, lacking the freedom to live their lives. They were groomed and recruited during their formative years, with a heavy trust held over their heads, as well as threats of poverty or ostracization from their family. Some of the most tragic and secret traffickers are family members and their victims appear to be well-paid executives or managers of the family business.

I want to help people understand that they are free. To recognize that we don't owe our families anything but respect and kindness. We do not have to pay with our lives for the lives that they have given us. After all we didn't ask to come here so why should we feel guilty and indebted. Please do not misunderstand me, I'm not seeking to encourage the villainization of our family members. Instead, I am simply encouraging that we stop deifying them.

It's our sacred responsibility to ourselves to humanize our family members, putting them in their proper place so that we might have an appropriate relationship with them. This allows us to set our sights and focus on the relationship we have with our Higher Power. Our connection to our Higher Power impacts our relationship with our highest self, which enables us to access our deepest desires and connect to our soul's purpose.

The most important relationship in our lives is our relationship with our Higher Power and ourselves. When we let go of unrealistic expectations of the finite and fallible human beings in our lives, and instead set or sights upon our infinite, benevolent creator, everything becomes possible. Healing, freedom, and the awakening of our soul's deepest desires, our true purpose. As long as we are distracted by codependent relationships where we're seeking validation externally, we remain trapped in our ego and disconnected from our divine identity.

If you have a goal or dream that you're committed to manifesting, and it has not yet come to fruition despite your best efforts, perhaps it's because of a limiting belief. In order for one's external reality to line up with their intentions, both the intention and the action must match the vibrational frequency of the desired outcome, and our vibrational frequency is deeply impacted by our beliefs.

Let's look at our subconscious mind which uses approximately 88% of our brain power to handle everything that our body needs to function properly. Within, it contains all the programs that control the way we think, what we believe, the way we feel, behave, and react. If our subconscious is operating on auto pilot, how do we go about taking control of it?

Our conscious and subconscious minds are in collaboration with each other. The job of our subconscious mind is to prove that our conscious mind is always right. If we consciously believe that we cannot be, do, or have something, then we are always going to be right.

Our subconscious mind will create the circumstances, selecting the perfect people to place in our lives to prove that we are right. So, how do we get into the driver's seat of our subconscious mind? Simple. We must go back to the Source.

Our thoughts and beliefs are not our original creation. Whatever beliefs or thoughts we have that are interfering with our confidence, self-esteem, and ability to attract the right opportunities and relationships into our lives, were developed during our most formative years before the age of eight. During that time, we absorbed the information surrounding us, from our family, cultural, and religious units, taking on the beliefs we experienced as our own. It's rare for a person to examine these core beliefs, but it's a critical and necessary process if we're going to try and transcend that which limits us.

I've found that when someone is struggling to shift a belief it's typically because shifting the belief would betray the system in which the belief was originated.

For example, I've worked with homosexual clients who struggled with their self-esteem and freedom. Somehow their family of origin, culture, or religion, had planted a message that it wasn't okay to be homosexual. As much as they disagree consciously, if they don't take the time to do the work to dismantle these beliefs at the core level, they will never be able to shift the belief.

In order to shift these beliefs, we have to ensure that we're not holding the person or institution from whom the belief originated on a pedestal so that they become a Higher Power in our life, which then impacts our decisions and beliefs. Think about it, if your parent is devoutly religious, it's an impossibility for you to defy their religion without defying your parent. Therefore, it's necessary that we demote our parent from Higher Power status so that we can separate our love and relationship to them from our commitments to ourselves, as well as separating ourselves from the religion or culture that will then provide us with the freedom to choose what we believe. And although our beliefs may offend or upset our family members, if we're not deifying them then we'll continue to have the freedom to adjust our relationships appropriately, without harming ourselves in the process.

It is possible to hold two separate emotions simultaneously. For example, you can love your culture or religion of origin, and yet not align with the beliefs, or maintain your membership or association with it. We don't have to change our religion or culture. We also don't have to fight against them. Instead, we can accept things for what they are, and choose to associate with them or not. The choice is always ours. Just because we come from somewhere, raised in a particular religion, we are never condemned to perpetually participate in that belief. Again, the choice is always ours. We're allowed to grow out of, up and away from, things that no longer serve us. This is our divine right as a sovereign human being. More than a right, it's our personal responsibility, to make the life choices that best serve us and who we choose to be.

It's no more right for us to try to change other people than for them to try to change us. I have the right to live my life, just as others have the right to live theirs. It's a part of our mission, our purpose, to align ourselves with that which serves and empowers us, walking away from that which does not, no matter how painful or uncomfortable it may be.

I've found both personally and professionally in relationship with my clients, so much unnecessary suffering when we are trying to hold onto ourselves and the past simultaneously when the past no longer serves us. When it no longer resonates with who we truly are.

Part of the evolution, maturation, and individuation of growing up means being able to walk away from that which no longer serves us and walk towards that which embodies our highest truth. We don't have to condemn something just because we no longer align with it. We can choose to love something from a distance. We can appreciate the way that it contributed to us in the past, as well as how it may have helped shape us, while simultaneously setting it aside and moving toward other things that will better empower our growth and evolution as we become who we truly wish to be.

So, what happens when we fail to individuate ourselves from our family systems? What happens when we stay stuck trying to live up to the image that someone else has created for us?

It's perfectly normal for a small child to be enmeshed with his or her family after all a child and their mother exist as a single ecosystem for the first year of life. The mother is the child's source of food, and the child's nervous system is regulating in concert with its mothers. The child is totally dependent upon their environment and the people in it to protect them, nurture them, and show them who to be.

However, we are supposed to learn from this and grow beyond it. The bird is not meant to stay in the nest forever. The day arrives when the little birdie flies away from the nest and creates its own.

When we stay stuck in infantile roles inside of dysfunctional family systems, all sorts of unhealthy paradigms emerge such as codependency and emotional incest.

Codependency is most simply defined as the act of allowing our feelings about ourselves to depend fully on how someone else feels about us, while emotional incest is most simply defined as a parent or guardian who is looking to a child to fulfill their emotional needs in inappropriate ways.

An example of emotional incest may be if an adult is parentifying their child, leaning upon them to provide advice, guidance, or support. It doesn't matter how mature or compassionate a 7-year-old child is, they are in no way qualified to provide marital advice, nor is it in any way appropriate for the troubles and frustrations of an adult marriage to be disclosed to an innocent child.

When a parent turns to a child for friendship or counseling, they damage the relationship. It's the job of the parent, to provide guidance and support to their child, not the other way around.

Little boys who are told that they are now the man of the house after a divorce, or their father's untimely death, shoulder an unbearable burden. Those little boys grow up to be quintessential lone rangers. They become men who are doomed to be the hero, feeling obligated and beholden to rescue damsels in distress. These boys often spend their lives feeling overly responsible, sacrificing themselves, and never feeling truly supported or loved.

Conversely mama's boys who are spoiled and infantilized by their mothers often suppress their masculinity, and independence. The price that a young man pays for surrendering to the comfort of his mother's coddling is castration which causes him to become anxious and neurotic. It costs him his natural leadership, independence, and strength as a man.

A young girl who has taken on the role of caring for her father never learns appropriate boundaries and will often sacrifice herself unnecessarily to care for others. She typically grows up being attracted to men who have mental health issues or struggle with substance abuse. She often finds herself feeling victimized by having to sacrifice herself to care for others.

Young girls who are spoiled by their fathers, raised to believe that they can do no wrong, and are princesses never having to pay for the consequences of their actions, who never have to pull their weight or fulfill responsibilities, will often leave their father's homes as entitled, narcissistic, self-centered, emotionally stunted girls who struggle to reach their potential as responsible women.

Now of course we are talking about extremes, and these are generalizations. It's impossible to capture in a single chapter or even in a single book all the many varying nuances of how these issues present themselves. The bottom line though is this — those individuals who've grown up within a dysfunctional family dynamic can find themselves somewhere on this spectrum, and the sooner they are able to discover the truth to themselves, committing to doing the work and healing, the sooner they will be free from it and able to move on to create a brighter future.

Judy Morris

Self-Esteem: Wholeness & Integrity

I was an only child and very lonely growing up. Being raised by elderly people who didn't have the energy or stamina to keep up with a young child combined with having a mother who was pre-occupied with working to provide for us, no father, and no siblings to hang out with (my brother didn't come along until I was 14), I was desperate for attention, affection, and connection. Any little crumb of attention that came my way I jumped on and became attached to the person offering it. I had very low self-esteem, which made me extremely vulnerable to participating in relationships that were unhealthy and co-dependent.

Once I got into recovery, I began to realize that the more I tried to prove my worth, the more I was affirming the opposite.

I always thought that in order to feel loved I needed to be loved by others. I had no idea about self-love or about self-esteem coming from esteemable acts. I thought that if others approved of me, paid attention to me, wanted me, loved me, and needed me, I would feel good about myself. And although there is no denying that it feels great to have connections with others and to be loved by others, we must also recognize that it becomes problematic if the person seeking those connections does not have a firm foundation of self-esteem to stand on independently.

If an insecure person seeks something outside themselves to feel ok, they will soon realize that putting their self-esteem in someone else hands is ill advised and creates an unsustainable dynamic. We have all known insecure people who are afraid to meet life on life's terms. People who are self-abandoning, never having learned how to care for themselves properly, so they continue to seek that care from others. They like to find a stronger person that they can depend on for guidance, protection, and affirmation. Disillusionment and increased helplessness are the result, because ultimately all their protectors either flee or die leaving them abandoned and once more alone, feeling even more insecure than they started.

Self-esteem comes from esteemable acts. Think about it. How do you feel about yourself when you are mean, selfish, lazy, or dishonest? Do you feel good, or do you feel bad?

Personal integrity comes from aligning our actions with our behaviors. For example, if I say that I want to improve my health, talking to my close friends or family to enlist their support, and taking action with my diet and exercise. I start making small changes, I create accountability by sharing my goals and asking for support, and within 24 hours of taking these actions, I'm already feeling better about myself. On the other hand, if I promise myself, I am going to eat better to improve my health and I do NOTHING, and keep finding myself at the donut shop, I am going to continue feeling badly about myself.

The same holds true with personal relationships. If all we do is take and never want to give, if we lie, cheat, or gossip, if we are mean, impatient, intolerant, if we behave dishonorably, we'll feel terrible about ourselves, and our relationships will suffer. All these behaviors do not build self-esteem, they erode it. Our culture of 'it's not a big deal,' is a lie. Everything we do, every thought we think is a very big deal. It is either leading to our success or our demise.

When our actions align with our behavior and our thoughts are on a higher plane, we become untouchable. We're less likely to fall prey to the highs and lows that come from the ferris wheel of co-dependency (high being when we're feeling liked, and lows when we're feeling disliked).

Let's consider an analogy. If someone told you that you were a giraffe, you wouldn't doubt your identity as a human being. You firmly and deeply know that you are not a giraffe, that it's impossible that you are a giraffe, and the fact that this person said such a thing to you would only make you doubt their sanity, not your humanity.

However, we don't possess this kind of confidence when people insult or criticize us. Anytime someone makes a disparaging comment about our beauty, talent, or intelligence, suddenly, we fear that we've been found out, our inherent insecurity creeps in and we question our worth. In essence, we believe that we are giraffes (*figuratively speaking*) which is ridiculous.

Although people can certainly behave like jerks and act out in hurtful ways, people cannot hurt (*disclaimer, I am not talking about physical injury*) us. Not really. It's never the circumstance that hurts us, but our interpretation of it. If someone lies to us or cheats on us the pain doesn't come from their behavior, it comes from the story we tell ourselves about why it happened, and our fear of whatever we thought we had with that person being damaged or taken away.

We say something to ourselves like: "*if I were enough, if they really loved me - if I was worthy, then they wouldn't have cheated on me.*" When in reality, the cheating doesn't reveal your worth or beauty, it's simply an indication of something missing in their character and your relationship. If they are willing to deal with whatever caused them to act out in such a disreputable way, and the two of you are willing to work on whatever is missing in the relationship that contributed to the breakdown of it, to begin with, then it can be resolved and healed without any damage to your sense of self. That doesn't mean that you won't feel sad or scared. But it doesn't have to shake your sense of self or your sense of value.

It's the same thing at work. If you're dealing with a challenge at work then there may be something to work on in your performance, a new skill to learn. But again, it has nothing to do with your inherent worth. The culture that we live in has perpetuated a belief that we are our successes or failures. Think about the way we language it, we don't say: "*I'm successful in my work*", or "*my work life is successful*," or "*my marriage is successful*" we say: "*I AM successful*," and we have the I AM connected to the success. Therefore, it only stands to reason that when we are no longer experiencing success in that area of our life - i.e., such as job loss, disability, or divorce, then it becomes "*I AM a failure.*" This connection that we make between our results and our worth is detrimental to our self-esteem and stability. Our results are indications of our behaviors and actions which are influenced by our thoughts and feelings, ALL of which can be improved upon. The danger of equating our results with our value is that we are then dependent upon people, places, and things that we are ultimately powerless over.

By giving our power away to external forces that we have no control over, we leave ourselves in a vulnerable position because it grants others permission to determine our value. When we confuse our results with our self-worth, we lose our stability, and become disconnected from the truth which is we are perfect, whole, and complete. However, if we are going to experience that truth, then our worth must be inherent and cannot be dependent upon anything outside of ourselves. This is a simple concept but difficult to implement in our daily lives.

The Shadow Side of Modern Culture

There are two sides to every story. The light side and the shadow side. And this does not just apply to personal psychology or spirituality. It applies to modern culture as well.

The light side of modern culture is freedom and increased equality for people. And, as if that were not enough, we have been given one of the biggest gifts — the internet, which has afforded us the ability to conduct business and personal relationships globally. It's added convenience to our lives by enabling us to have hundreds of books on a small tablet as well as being able to research any subject at any hour on our laptop or handheld device. Having smartphones to order a Lyft instead of having to call a Taxi, we can place an order for a meal or groceries to be quickly delivered, we have on-line stores available 24/7 to be able to order and ship a gift at any hour of the day or night. Anything and everything we could ever desire, seems to be available at the touch of a button.

But all that freedom and convenience also has a shadow side. There has never been a time in modern history where we have had more access to education, information, or services. We have choices to work remotely or in a traditional office environment. To remain single or to get married. But one of the shadows of choice is analysis paralysis. Sometimes, with so many choices we find ourselves obsessed with making the right one. In addition, we get seduced by one of the greatest challenges of growing up in western culture, the idea that something outside of ourselves will make us happy.

We who have been raised in or have lived in western culture for any length of time have been fed a steady stream of marketing campaigns and advertisements of various kinds, all telling us that the road to happiness lies in looking younger, more attractive, and driving a fancier car (especially if you live in Los Angeles). We need to make more money, have a fancier title, a better education, a bigger bank account, or a lower number on the scale. Our lives have become filled with 'If only" statements. If only we could be better looking, or more successful, or richer, or more educated. If only we had better partners, if only our families had given us more advantages, etc. the list goes on and on.

We are inundated with a constant stream of endless cries for our attention whether they be on social media platforms or magazines in line at the grocery store. Every which way we turn there is external stimuli that is trying to tell us that we too can achieve happiness if only we have some external materialistic thing to make us more or better. This has perpetuated the lie that we need something man-made, chemically produced to enhance our lives. Is it any wonder with this kind of message that we are so lonely, so unhappy, so depressed, so filled with anxiety?

Is it any surprise that we are in an addiction crisis such as the world has never seen? That we live in a world where it is statistically more likely for a person in the USA to die of an opiate overdose than in a car crash!

Is it any wonder that Americans are medicating themselves with alcohol, marijuana, and pills just to get through the day? How many memes do we see on our social media feeds that joke about that desperately needed glass of wine at the end of the day? Is it really a joke or is it simply the tragic reality of living lives so unfulfilling and stressful that we need to chemically escape from them?

The problem here cannot be solved by a makeover or a promotion. This is a problem of the spiritual variety and requires a spiritual solution.

We have lost the connection to our divinity perhaps because Madison Avenue and Wall Street have objectified us. They have convinced us that we are no longer people to be loved, or families to raise. We have become objects to be improved, and problems to be solved.

We must wake up from this untruth. We must untangle ourselves from this web of marketing and consumerism. We desperately need to find ourselves, our inherent value, and our self-worth. We need to connect with our Higher Power and the Universe. We need to connect to each other, not just on a screen but face to face, looking into each other's eyes, embracing one another, experiencing love and connection.

When we are deeply connected to our divinity and our wholeness there is no need for something outside of ourselves to fix us, prop us up, or make us feel better. We move from needing people and things in from a needy co-dependent place to sharing ourselves with others and connecting with others from a place of contributing and being contributed to.

When we come from a place of wholeness our foibles are no longer detrimental but a part of our humanity - opportunities for growth and learning. When we are coming from a place of wholeness, we can see the wounds that need healing, addictions that need recovery, and any other number of areas of our lives that we need to set straight, without diminishing our worth.

Pause for a moment and imagine relating to your problems as just that, problems to be solved, not that you are a problem. We have enmeshed ourselves within our circumstances. We don't say: *"I have a success"* we say: *"I am successful".* Too often we say, *"I am a failure"* instead of *"I have a failed endeavor."*

We have things, illnesses, and challenges that we deal with, but these do not add to or diminish our worth. When we fully concede to our innermost self that we are inherently worthy because we are children of the Universe, emanations of the divine, then at that moment we begin to grasp the truth of being and take an important step toward liberating our souls.

It never ceases to amaze me that we spend hundreds of thousands of dollars on education for careers. We spend thousands of hours studying engineering or architecture or design. We spend so much time to learn our craft, to make a living, but we never learn how to make a life. We don't spend very much time learning about ourselves, the Universe that we live in, or how to create fulfilling relationships. If someone is experiencing a challenge in their career, they receive coaching, feedback, additional education. But if they are dealing with a challenge in their relationship or their family, they're more likely to get a divorce then to go to therapy. How easily we give up on our families, our children, and our marriages, and how fervently we cling to the almighty dollar in our careers. Our priorities have gotten completely confused. We are so profoundly out of balance as human beings that we've lost any sense of connection to the divine. The sense of being a person among people or a neighbor among neighbors. We've become completely polarized by political disagreements and the levels of violence within our communities has risen to record levels. What is the source of all of this?

A man can only know another man to the extent that he knows himself. We cannot meet anyone else on a deeper level than we have met our own self. If we have not invested in our own development as a human being, our own spiritual exploration, if we don't understand how we are connected to everything and everyone in this world, then of course we feel separate, and that separation only fuels our egos. The ego is very cleverly designed to protect itself, defend its position, and destroy anything that opposes it.

Bronnie Ware, an Australian nurse who spent several years caring for patients throughout the last 12 weeks of their lives, recorded many of those individuals' dying epiphanies within her book, *The Top Five Regrets of the Dying*.

Those five regrets, as witnessed by Ware are:

- *"I wish I'd had the courage to live a life true to myself, not the life others expected of me."*
- *"I wish I hadn't worked so hard."*
- *"I wish I'd had the courage to express my feelings."*
- *"I wish I had stayed in touch with my friends."*
- *"I wish that I had let myself be happier."*

What would your biggest regret be if this was your last day of life? Knowing that fulfillment comes from knowing who you are, being free, being fully self-expressed, and not the commercially promoted shiny objects being advertised, what would you do today to foster healing, health, sobriety, and recovery? How would you invest in your relationship with yourself and others?

When I'm working with clients who seem to be stuck and struggling with or resisting doing the work to free and heal themselves, it's often the fear that their attempts will not work that keep them from even starting.

Many people have a fear or superstition that somehow there is something inherently broken, unhealable, or irredeemable in them, and if they go into the process of doing the work that is only going to uncover and confirm their fatal flaw.

This is the ultimate myth! THERE IS NOTHING WRONG WITH YOU! If we're able to start relating to ourselves as eternal, spiritual beings that are having a human experience, seeing ourselves as being perfectly designed, understanding that all the challenges we've been faced with are part of our evolution, and that life is not an achievement but an experience, then our challenges can occur as just that, challenges that we're dealing with. Challenges that hold no indication of our worth or lack thereof.

I've had the privilege of working with people who have serious, debilitating disabilities like cerebral palsy, and I have seen them live purposeful and fulfilled lives. You don't need a perfect mind or a perfect body to have a purposeful and fulfilled life. All that is required is radical honesty, humility, and a willingness to do the work to achieve your highest potential.

If we continue to honor false beliefs and superstitions, then we'll continue to get those same results. I remember a dear friend shared with me an epiphany she had during her struggle in recovery. She stated that she had an 'aha' moment one day in treatment when it occurred to her that she had been fiercely loyal to her addiction. She pondered what would happen if she shifted that fierce loyalty to her recovery instead. Her theory worked. At the time of my writing this book, she has over three years of sobriety. What would be possible for you, if you shifted your fierce loyalty away from your false beliefs and superstitions, and instead focused on recovery from whatever chains bind you?

As stated earlier, I've worked with individuals who have significant disabilities and I've seen people with severe cerebral palsy bound to their wheelchairs yet still living meaningful, purposeful, and successful lives with fulfilling romantic relationships and careers.

A phenomenal example of this is Stephen Hawking. Here's someone who while wheelchair-bound refused to allow his physical limitations to dull his genius. He soared academically and scientifically, making incredible contributions to society. He enjoyed fulfilling relationships with his family and married despite his physical challenges. The misinformation, the myth that our circumstances are what has all the power must be broken for us to step into our own power. I'm not diminishing the fact that people who come from more compromised backgrounds will often have a more difficult time achieving their goals. But that doesn't mean it's impossible.

I've included a brief list below, shining a light on some of individuals I find to be most inspiring. All individuals who were at extreme disadvantage, yet not only fulfilled their goals, but exceeded them. If we want to accomplish something the only thing standing between us and that which we desire is our willingness to pursue it and make the necessary changes to achieve it. Now, you might look at this list and think, *"those are all geniuses, but I'm nobody."* Remember, you are exactly who you say you are. If you say that you're nobody then that is exactly who you will be, but the opposite is also true. If you say that you are brilliant and capable, then you will spark your brilliance and begin producing amazing results towards that which is meaningful to you. I encourage you to look to this list as inspiration NOT comparison.

Pay attention to any similarities you might find, between your own background, passion, and purpose and those of the individuals on this list, but do not compare. There is no one else like you in the entire Universe. You are uniquely skilled to fulfill whatever passion is in your heart. If you will only let your passion guide you toward your true purpose you will find the courage to heal, the curiosity to learn and grow, and the fortitude to act and produce.

Judy Morris

Inspiring Individuals

- Bill Wilson
- Abraham Lincoln
- Harriet Tubman
- Walt Disney
- Tony Robbins
- Jack Canfield
- Steven Hawking
- Temple Grandin
- The Wright Brothers
- Henry Ford
- YOU

Moving From Victim to Authority in Your Own Life

Alignment. Our actions, behavior, and speech must all align with our commitments, dreams, and goals.

Perhaps it seems obvious, but too often it isn't. One of the most self-sabotaging behaviors people have is behaving incongruently with their commitment's dreams and goals. A simple example is someone who joins a gym and says that they're committed to their health and vitality. Months go by, and they haven't attended a single class, nor have they stepped foot in the gym. Instead, they've spent their evenings and weekends eating junk food and watching television. They are practicing couch potatoes.

But, if you happen to get into a conversation with them about it, they'll tell you something along the lines of they're having realized they just aren't a gym person, or that the gym doesn't work for them. Nonsense! If we step back and look more closely at the above excuses, we see that the purchase of a gym membership never promised magical inspiration. Purchasing a membership does not provide or instill motivation into a person. The membership exists as a tool, access to a structure, a place to go for community and support, a place to empower your goal. Part of self-honesty, awareness, and becoming responsible for our lives includes looking at where we're dissatisfied, depressed, and unfulfilled, as well as being brutally honest with ourselves about where we've been lying to ourselves. Where our behaviors and actions are inconsistent with what we say it as we want. Until we have the courage and integrity to admit our own self-sabotage and do the work to align ourselves with our deepest desires, we will continue to perpetuate a life of failure and disappointment.

Let's talk about another myth. The myth of motivation. There seems to be a culturally widespread belief that motivation is a requirement of action. This is false.

For example, picture a cold dark room. You're fast asleep, and it's 4 o'clock in the morning. It's freezing outside, and suddenly, you're woken up by the sound of your dog scratching at the door because they need to go outside. You don't have to be motivated to get out of bed and take your dog outside, you may not want to do it, it may be incredibly uncomfortable, but you do it anyway because you love your pet and because you're committed to not having your pet defecate on your beautiful hardwood floor or carpet. Your commitment is to your pet and to the cleanliness and beauty of your home. Those are the driving factors.

Most people don't realize that what they're really committed to is the easy way out. We are more interested in being comfortable and playing it safe, then fulfilling our dreams and goals. When we get real with ourselves and tell the truth, that it's been flat out laziness or fear that's kept us frozen in a Groundhog Day of junk food and Netflix, in that staggering and sobering moment we realize that we are the only person who has been standing in the way of our dreams.

As Marie Forleo so eloquently says: *"instead of saying I don't have the time, say I haven't been willing to make the time".*

You may be thinking is there no exception to this rule? What about people that are suffering from physical ailments or mental health issues? People that are dealing with mental or physical health issues have an added challenge to deal with. But now the question becomes what is the person doing about their mental or physical health issue? I've seen people complaining of their diabetic condition and yet continuing to consume excessive amounts of soda pop, processed foods, alcohol, and sugar. If we're committed to fulfilling our goals and dreams and we have mental or physical health issues, then we must first and foremost deal with those things. If we have an addiction, we need to get into recovery. If we're diabetic, we need to get that stabilized and improve our habits. We must ask ourselves if we have done everything possible to restore our wellness with whatever conditions we're dealing with, then once we're stabilized, we can move forward in the next step toward our goal.

When I say stabilized, I don't mean perfect. We must accept that we are all perfectly imperfect. We cannot expect to be perfect in an imperfect world. Perfectionism is a sickness that doesn't allow us to embrace our own humanity. The first step within the 12-steps is powerlessness. In AA the step says: *"We admitted we were powerless over alcohol – that our lives had become unmanageable."* To gain power over my own alcoholism, I had to first admit my powerlessness over alcohol. Powerlessness is paradoxical in nature. The moment we accept our powerlessness over alcohol is the moment we gain our power over alcohol. Not power to drink it, power not to drink it. You see the more we try to exert power over that which we have no power the more unmanageable our life becomes. The fact that I have alcoholism means that I cannot successfully drink. The more I resisted this fact, the more I tried to prove otherwise (that I could control my drinking which I could not) the more I had to keep drinking. My resistance perpetuated the problem. The moment I admitted my powerlessness over alcohol I no longer had to drink. When I accepted the truth about myself and my inability to process alcohol like a "normal" person I was able to stop drinking which opened the door to my recovery.

Powerlessness is an important concept that people do not like to talk about in our society. In fact, quite the opposite, we are obsessed with power. We are obsessed with something that we don't fully understand. There are things we have power over and things that we are powerless over. We are powerless over people, places, and things. We cannot control anyone or anything. The only person we have control over is ourselves. So, in the example with my own alcoholism, I am powerless over the fact that I have the disease of alcoholism, but I am not powerless over what I am going to do about it. I am not powerless over my ability to heal from it. And healing doesn't mean regaining the ability to drink. It means maintaining my ability to not drink. I am powerless over my height (unless I put on a pair of high heels), but I am not powerless over my relationship to my height. I am powerless over the family system I was born into and any childhood trauma that I experienced, but I am not powerless over what I do about it. I can go to therapy, read books, educate myself, and take actions toward my own healing. I am powerless over the maladaptive coping mechanisms I created to survive, but I am not powerless over learning new ones that are healthier. If a person is born with a disability (visual/hearing impairment, etc.) they are powerless over having that disability, but they are not powerless over who they are going to be in the face of it, they are not powerless over learning how to adapt in healthy ways and making the best of their lives under the circumstances. Understanding what we have power over and what we do not is an important discernment to have to live a fulfilled life that is deeply grounded in reality.

It doesn't matter what limitations you have. If we accept our limitations with self-compassion and let go of the jealousy/anger/disappointment that our life looks different than what we may have wanted, the seemingly impossible becomes possible.

Allow me to introduce you to Bill Porter. Born in San Francisco, California, in 1932, Bill moved to Portland, Oregon with his mother at a young age. He graduated high school in the 1950's a time when America was not friendly to those who were disabled. He wanted to work very badly and went to great lengths to obtain a job but was unsuccessful due to the highly discriminatory environment of the time. Employers didn't have to provide a reasonable accommodation to employees until The Americans with Disabilities Act (ADA) was signed into law on July 26, 1990.

Before then there were no enforceable guidelines for employers regarding people who were disabled. Bill had cerebral palsy. He had a speech impediment and although he was not restricted to a wheelchair, he did have trouble walking. It was recommended that Bill apply to receive disability, but he refused. Mr. Porter eventually convinced Watkins Incorporated to give him a position as a door-to-door salesman, selling their products on a seven-mile route in the Portland area. Pause for a moment and think about that. This is a man with challenges walking, and a noticeable speech impediment, who took on a 7-mile route to sell items door-to-door during which he would be speaking primarily with strangers. Not only did Watkins Incorporated hire Bill for the position, but he went on to become their top salesman and worked for the company for over forty years.

Allow me to introduce you to another extraordinary individual - Rick Hoyt, a quadriplegic who also has cerebral palsy. Rick has spent his whole life in a wheelchair but didn't allow that to stop him from fulfilling his dream of participating in marathons. Rick's father, Dick Hoyt, in order to help his son's dreams, come true, pushed him in a specialized wheelchair through dozens of Boston Marathons and hundreds of other races. When we look at Team Hoyt, we're able to see how a family can face seemingly insurmountable challenges by being willing to use their creativity, resourcefulness, and faith in what's possible rather than what was predictable. Being willing to live in that space, in the space of creativity, resourcefulness, and faith, that is where the magic happens.

Dick Hoyt was an average guy, he wasn't an athlete, but he became one because that's what his son's dream was asking of him. His own dream as a father was to help his son have as normal of a life as possible, thus he chose to answer the call and become an athlete himself. He was willing to go to any length, showing that where there is a will there is away.

What makes someone like Bill Porter or Rick Hoyt see the world as their oyster vs. their enemy? It's not because they are in a more advantaged place. Quite the opposite. But the advantage that both these men exhibit is in their perspective. They don't see life from their limitation, they see it from their capability. They focus on what they can do vs. what they cannot.

Let's talk about the power of perspective. Perspective the old "Glass Half Full Scenario." The glass is also half empty.

This may sound like a cliché, but it's also very powerful. The glass, in and of itself, doesn't give the person holding on to it, their sense of experience. Their own personal perspective does.

The person viewing the glass as half full is grateful for what they have. The person with a half empty glass probably feels upset, maybe even cheated.

It's the same situation, but from a different perspective. Neither are the absolute truth, and yet both are real for the person holding the glass.

With awareness, we realize that a simple shift in our own perspective gives us an entirely new experience of ourselves and the landscapes of our lives.

This is me, my height, my ethnic background, my ancestral lineage, and the trauma that comes with it, my socio-economic upbringing, my culture, and foundational education. These are all things that are facts of my life. These are unchangeable. I must not only learn to see them from a fresh perspective, but I must also accept myself and my story fully and whole heartedly to make peace and to move forward toward my future with a sense of purpose vs. struggle. You see, if I do not accept myself, my life, and my story, I will pursue relationships, careers, from a place of being incomplete, to fix or change something about me which will never lead me to my purpose or fulfillment. I must move toward my goals from a place of wholeness otherwise I am just a victim looking to be rescued, going to any length to get my needs met at the expense of others.

Acceptance is the answer to ALL my problems. Acceptance gets a bad rap and is totally misunderstood. Most people think that if they accept something, then they are condoning it, or saying that it was "okay." That's inaccurate. To accept something is simply to recognize it as true. That which already is. It doesn't mean that we've asked for it, wanted it, or like it. It simply means that we're acknowledging what has already happened and are being honest about it.

If you only have a high school diploma, or are divorced, disabled, or are now 20 years older than you thought you'd be and still working an entry level job, then those are the facts.

Going back to the glass half empty analogy, you can either dwell on what has already transpired, which you can do nothing about, and suffer over what might have been, or you can get real and think about what you do have.

Such as passion, enthusiasm, and hard-won experience. Or something new, different, and powerful to contribute to the world.

When we focus on our strengths, rather than our weaknesses, we're able to see more clearly what we bring to the table and start moving towards our goals.

Being aware of the facts, and accepting ourselves the way that we are, and the way that we are not, opens the door to authenticity.

Judy Morris

"Always be a first-rate version of yourself and not a second-rate version of someone else." - Judy Garland

Authenticity is defined as being real or genuine, not copied, or false. This is a crucial element of successfully manifesting our deepest desires. To attract the career opportunities and relationships that are best for us, we must be ourselves. If we are pretending to be someone else, then we attract the life that is a fit for the person we're pretending to be and will never experience fulfillment in that life because it isn't meant for us.

Fantasy Island

The most painful part of being a child was the powerlessness of it. Not having a say in any matter. Authority figures held the power to dismantle my entire world by getting divorced and bringing their new partner and their children into the equation. Moving, changes in job schedule, and work demands. All these things were incredibly impactful, and I never got a vote on any of them

The instability was maddening, and I made a promise to myself that I would NEVER be powerless like that again. I would pave my own path and make my own decisions. NO ONE would toss me about EVER again.

All that said, you can understand that I was in a hurry to grow up because I wanted POWER. Power over my life, my surroundings, my circumstances, my relationships. However, the unfavorable circumstances in my life were unfolding at speeds faster than my natural aging process. I knew that I needed to figure out another way to escape. After all, I grew up in Hollywood, the land of make-believe. People come to Los Angeles from all over the world to reinvent themselves. As a native who grew up around the entertainment industry, I knew all about pretend. So, what was I waiting for?! I didn't like certain facts about myself or my life, so I made up new ones. For example, I didn't like my age, so I told people I was older. I wanted to be around people with power and influence, so I surrounded myself with older friends. I became the embodiment of the persona that I invented.

I'll never forget the first time I ordered a drink in a bar. I was with my boyfriend at the time, and his family at a very elegant and expensive Japanese restaurant. I was a little nervous having dinner with his family for the first time. But this was it, I had successfully landed my older man, we

49

were together, and I was accepted. Everyone adored me. More importantly, everyone believed me. He was 28 and I was 15, although he believed me to be 22.

I knew exactly what I needed to calm my nerves. I could see the elaborate bar in the distance, across the room from our table. I excused myself for a moment and made my way down the three steps that lead from the dining room into the bar. The bar itself was empty, except for the bartender who was putting away glasses and cutting limes. That was the moment of truth. I knew I could not fail. I could no longer think of this as pretending, I had to be the woman that I wanted to be. I had to believe it myself in every fiber of my being. I had to order that drink with the confidence and surety that would pass a polygraph test. I would not be questioned; I would not be carded.

I didn't miss a beat as I clutched my red suede wallet, prepared to pay for the drink before it was even ordered. I walked confidently up to the bar, head held high, determined - I looked her straight in the eye and said, *"Good evening, I'd like a vodka tonic please."* I rolled my eyes and said it's been one of those days, she nodded in agreement. I went on to complain about the stress in the office, how it's never ending, and how being a legal secretary was so very demanding. My boss was a taskmaster and extremely difficult to deal with. We chatted about my imaginary job as she made my drink. I tipped her generously as I clutched my drink, taking a few sips before returning to the dinner table.

If I thought I had arrived before, it was truly solidified in that moment. I felt invincible, in control, powerful, on top of the world. There are no words to describe to you what that moment gave to me, how it convinced me that make-believe was possible, and that I could transcend my circumstances by pretending my way out of them.

I met Marco on a sunny August afternoon. He was a friend of a friend. Truth be told, my friend had a crush on him, and she'd enlisted my help in being her wing-woman, since I was far more persuasive than she. I didn't mind playing the part of Cyrano de Bergerac minus the cloak and dagger. However, our little plan took a turn in the wrong direction. Marco informed me that he wasn't interested in my friend, she wasn't his type and therefore my attempts were useless. He then proceeded to tell me that I was exactly his type.

I was conflicted. I'd only spoken with Marco over the phone, so I couldn't understand how he knew that I was his type. He informed me that he'd seen me at an event we'd both attended. He already had the upper hand. I was also concerned about how my friend going to feel, knowing that she had lustful feelings for Marco, but his interest was in me. I met Marco at the next party we both attended, and it was clear after a few moments of talking, that there was an unmistakable connection between us. The chemistry was palpable. He was exactly what I needed. He was sexy, fun, successfully employed, drove a beautiful car, and was crazy about me. I broke the news to my friend. I told her that Marco just wasn't interested in her, and I asked why I should suffer by rejecting his advances, when he wasn't going to be with her anyway? To me, it was perfectly acceptable. They had never dated, and he wasn't interested in her, so I wasn't really interfering in anything. Although my friend was hurt at first and unhappy with my decision, she eventually accepted it and moved on.

Creating my own fantasy island to reside on with Marco started out great. It didn't matter that it started out with a lie. I lied to him about my age.

It was so easy. I was getting what I wanted and navigating the world by spinning my own intricate web of lies. Considering how much I was drinking during that time of my life, being intoxicated made it even easier. I justified my behavior by assuring myself that I wasn't stealing money or "hurting" anyone. I was just presenting myself as something different than who I was.

About a year into our relationship, Marco proposed to me. I was flabbergasted. We had talked about getting married, but I hadn't anticipated that we would get engaged so quickly. He was so happy. He would always tell me that the world was our oyster.

It all seemed logical, but the typical elation was missing for me. I didn't realize it at the time, but I was terrified of being with Marco forever. As much as I cared for him and enjoyed our relationship for what it was, deep down I knew that he wasn't my forever. However, I didn't have high enough self-awareness or esteem, or the courage to be honest with myself. All I knew was survival. And maintaining my relationship with Marco was a survival tactic, although I would not have recognized it as such at the time.

The problem with living in a fantasy world is that we create a mask for ourselves to hide behind and then attract a match for that mask. Living inauthentically comes at a very high price and the bill comes without warning at a late and inconvenient date.

You see, like attracts like, and water seeks its own level. I wasn't the only one with a secret. Marco had his own secret. He had a drug problem that he hid from me. I was a highly functioning alcoholic, and he was a highly functioning drug addict. We were a perfect match.

I had created a character based on fear, fueled by ego. I was pretending to be a devil-may-care young woman of the world. I was flirtatious, entertaining, and charming, sometimes too much so. Men flocked to me like moths to a flame. And I had no qualms about using my feminine wiles to get what I wanted and what I wanted was attention. My careless behavior led me into many compromising situations, and I ended up hurting Marco. But I didn't care, I justified it because he had hurt me with his sprees, disappearing for days. I may have been dating other men occasionally behind his back, but he was cheating too, his mistress just happened to be a white powder.

This inauthentic life came at a price.

It cost me my youth. I was already a parentified child who basically skipped childhood and moved straight into being a teenager, and then a fiancée by the time I was 16 ½. I was telling one set of people that I was 18 and another set that I was 22 and didn't pause to consider the emotional ramifications of that.

By the time I did turn 18 I had a serious breakdown. It was no wonder. I had crushed my spirit under the pressures of the role I had created for myself, and the denial of the losses that I was grieving. You see, it was easier to pretend that I was all grown up and independent and that the abandonment, neglect, and loss that I had experienced as a child didn't matter. I couldn't bear the weight of the reality of it. That combined with the looming possibility of marriage which I was not prepared to step into, sent me over the edge.

I had wanted to go to college. I wanted to be a lawyer. But I didn't have the emotional or financial resources to accomplish either of those dreams. I had given up on my dreams. I couldn't afford them. I had fantasies instead. I plotted my escape from the circumstances of my life that I found unacceptable. I was a survivor, an escape artist. I didn't make choices based on desire, I made choices based on need. For example, when it came to men, what did they have that I needed and what did I have that they needed? If I needed you, I would become whoever you needed me to be. Being a Chamaeleon is dangerous. I got so busy taking on new roles that I lost myself in the process. Did I really like basketball or

Judy Morris

was I just pretending to because you did? It took a long time to wake up to myself.

"Ignoring who you truly, authentically are can literally be killing you... Forcing yourself to be someone you are not or stuffing down who you really are...will tax you so much that it will shorten your life by years and years"

- Phillip C. McGraw PhD

The Silent Threat of Deceiving Oneself

Experiencing a fulfilled life of vibrant health and self-expression requires that we break free from our masks, from our past, and that we be willing to wake up from the haze of denial, disassociation, and inauthenticity. This is what it takes to become aware. The first step toward freedom is awareness, and awareness starts with getting present to the facts.

No story and no judgment about where you are, or where you have been.

We cannot alter something that we are unaware of. If we don't know what the problem is, then we cannot find an appropriate solution. The driving force behind seeking a correct diagnosis, the only reason to attempt to understand the problem at hand, is not to berate or blame ourselves, to feel bad about ourselves or our circumstances. The purpose of this understanding is to become aware of what we're dealing with so that we can do something about it.

Think about it, if someone has an illness like cancer, a lack of awareness can mean the difference between life and death. The earlier an illness is caught, or diagnosed, the quicker it can be stopped, before it ravages the body. While it's difficult to admit that we have an addiction, it's difficult to admit that we struggle with a learning disability, it's difficult to admit that we have a mental health issue, it's something we must do. I get it, I experienced many of my own struggles when I had to come to my own admission of my alcoholism, depression, and other challenges/limitations. However, the freedom that came from the awareness combined with the willingness to take full responsibility for both my disease and my recovery was life changing. Once I stepped out of denial and into the reality of my situation, I was finally able to do something about it.

Part of becoming a sovereign, autonomous, individual is radical self-honesty which leads to awareness. We must be willing to embrace and understand our limitations to move past them. As long as we are pretending something, as long as we are unwilling to tell the truth, we'll remain stuck exactly where we are.

Here's a ridiculous but simple metaphor - imagine that you're in Newark New Jersey, and you want to go to Hawaii, but you feel ashamed that you're in Newark. So, you tell your driver that you're in New York City. Your driver would never be able to find you, pick you up, or help you get to the airport and then Hawaii. To get where we're going, we must know where we are. I warned you, that was going to be a silly example, but how absurd do we behave in our own lives when we pretend something that keeps us stuck. Dishonesty prevents us from understanding the true problem at hand which then conceals the actions required to get to the next point on our destination.

We all have opinions and interpretations about why things are the way they are and how we got to where we are now, in this moment. That is not the problem. The problem is that we think our opinion is fact. An opinion is not a fact, but one of many possible viewpoints, of any situation. The autopilot default stance that people take when they are experiencing failure, a failure to perform, a failure to achieve their goals, is to look for who is to blame. There are those that blame themselves and get weighed down in a messy bog of guilt and shame which doesn't foster learning, correction, or growth. Or they look for someone or something to blame which again doesn't foster learning, correction, or growth, in fact, it's worse, it places the individual in a victim stance. A victim of circumstance. You see it's not possible to be both empowered and a victim simultaneously. We are one or the other. We are either a victim, powerless over the unfair circumstances that are being thrown at us or we are the author of our life, fully responsible for the results or lack thereof and not from a victim place but from a place of ownership and full responsibility.

Let's talk about responsibility in more detail. Responsibility has a bad reputation. People generally associate it with a burden, blame, or obligation. And although one could associate responsibility to those words, that would most probably be the victim's interpretation. A victim would see responsibility as something put upon them, a burden that they must endure. A victim wouldn't see themselves as the cause of the circumstance at hand, they wouldn't see themself as the author of the circumstance or of their life.

Merriam Webster's Dictionary defines responsibility as the state of being the person who caused something to happen...reliability and trustworthiness.

Those are powerful words describing a powerful being. Something we often overlook when it comes to responsibility it that it also implies authority. We are the one who has the say as to how this is going to go. You see if we are responsible for the outcome, then we are responsible for the problem, which then also makes us responsible for the solution.

Whenever we assign blame to a person, place, or thing, we are giving our power away to that person, place, or thing, and rendering ourselves powerless. That renders us at the mercy of that person place or thing, leaving us as a mere spectator in the game of our life.

As tempting as it may seem at times to shrink and assign blame, I am no longer willing to do that. I no longer see responsibility as something to be feared or a burden to bear. I see it for what it is, the most precious and golden opportunity for me to be the author of my own life, the star, the hero of my own story.

Suffering comes from ignorance not from unfavorable circumstances. Another myth perpetuated in our western culture is that our circumstances dictate our happiness or lack thereof.

We truly believe that if we have unfavorable circumstances such as poverty, abuse, mental health issues, disabilities, or other challenges it's impossible for us to be happy?

We blame our pain, depression, addiction, and self-sabotage on the circumstances, the unhealthy codependent relationships, the lack of education etc. and although such circumstances may have made our assent toward our goals more challenging, it does not make it impossible.

We are not responsible for our trauma, we are not responsible for inherited limitations such as a disability, but we are responsible for our healing, and we are responsible for making the best of our circumstances.

The Cost of Inauthenticity

Another aspect of our lives that we need to bring awareness to is our culture. We live and work in a culture that prizes material wealth, prestige, and power as being paramount to happiness. And yet, how many of those materially wealthy, prestigious, and powerful people do we see who are struggling with unhappiness and failure in their personal lives? We live in a time in history when we have access to MORE of everything we could possibly imagine, and the result is not increased happiness. In pursuit of our culturally imposed values, we've lost our connection to our own values, our dreams, desires, and authenticity. It breaks my heart when I hear a college-bound person say: *"I hate finance, but I am headed to Wall Street as that is where the money is".* People are chasing dollar signs instead of pursuing their passion and it comes at a cost. When skill is traded for money void of any desire or personal connection it becomes a form of prostitution. We objectify ourselves and others, becoming nothing more that commodities for sale. No wonder we're so void of fulfillment and meaning in our careers. In addition to all this focus on the all-mighty dollar people we often live far away from our family of origin and are not affiliated with a spiritual community or humanitarian efforts, giving us all the more time and reason to focus on work and material success. We've forgotten how to dream, how to value ourselves, and each other. We've forgotten how magical it is to collaborate, connect, and create together. We've forgotten that success follows authentic self-expression. I invite you to set aside everything that society, our culture and even your family of origin has taught you about success and look within.

Let's take this example even further. I cannot tell you how many times I've worked with people we were unhappy at work but were afraid to leave.

59

Or maybe they enjoyed the company/people they worked with but hated the work/profession.

How we do one thing is how we do everything. So, chances are if you're unhappy at work then you're unhappy in your life. Sadly, this is far more prevalent than you may think. In a 2022 survey conducted by RealEstateWitch.com, it was found that nearly 60% of workers feel *some* negative emotions about their job, with nearly 1 in 4 feeling *only* negative emotions.

A significant portion of our country is unhappy at work and that makes for unhappy communities. Whenever I encounter someone who's rude or inconsiderate, I often wonder, does that person feel disrespected, unfulfilled, and stressed out at work?

Considering that we spend 40 plus hours per week at our jobs, it's an overwhelming amount of time to spend doing something that we're at best, neutral about, or at worst, that we dislike.

Why are we willing to spend years and years of our precious lives engaged in soul-crushing, unfulfilling roles? We try to minimize the impact of our choices by justifying them based on economic necessity or lack of opportunity in our geographic area, or due to lack of skill, experience, and education to pursue a different opportunity. There are many reasons we have for making compromises. However, what we're overlooking is the catastrophic long-term effects of such compromises. One of my favorite definitions of compromise is in Merriam Webster's Dictionary which states, to compromise is to cause the impairment of exposure to suspicion, discredit, or mischief.

We've all heard the premise that poor habits compromise poor health and reputation. The same holds true when we compromise our integrity and remain employed in a profession, or within an organization, that isn't in alignment with our dreams and desires. We become impaired; we discredit ourselves to ourselves.

Often, we become bound by golden handcuffs. We start making so much money that we're afraid we won't be able to replicate our salary in another position or company. It's important that we remember, we are priceless and there is no amount of money that can compensate for time spent away from our family, the stress, lack of work/life balance, personal satisfaction or the potential health issues that often accompany our unhappiness at work.

I've included below four reasons that you need to make a change. The sooner, the better!

- **Your Mental Health** — Being unhappy at work can take a serious toll on your mental health. Think about how irritability, depression, anxiety, OCD, and workaholism impact our moods. How many people fall prey to substance abuse (going home and drowning your sorrows in alcohol or other substances or popping uppers at work just to get through another boring and miserable day). Also, if you're in recovery from substance abuse, please note that being unhappy at work can often be linked to relapse. And nothing is worth risking your recovery.

- **Your Physical Health** — Unhappiness has been linked to depression which can compromise our immune system, leaving us fatigued and prey to obesity which is linked to heart disease.

- **Chronic Stress** — If you're in a demanding job with high levels of responsibility and deadlines, you could be in for more than a promotion. Chronic stress can increase your risk of heart attack and stroke. Stress reduction is critical to creating a state of emotional balance and a sense of well-being. It's impossible to have a sense of well-being if you hate your job.

- **Insomnia** — Unhappiness, depression, and chronic stress can lead to insomnia which in turn create serious health issues. Not getting enough sleep impairs judgement, motivation, reaction time, short-term memory, and even vision.

Marriage and family are undoubtedly important and incredibly rewarding, yet when we add the heavy burden of an unhappy work situation to familial obligations, life can become overwhelming. It can become more and more difficult to meet demands. How can we possibly give to our loved ones when our own cup is empty? How patient will we be when we walk through the door after 8 hours of demands, negativity, and doing something we hate? If we're exhausted at the end of the day, will we feel like going to the gym (self-care) or doing chores like stopping at the store for healthy meal choices? Probably not. Coming home depleted and unhappy is not a recipe for a happy family life. How frisky and romantic can we feel after a day of sedentary drudgery?

Self-esteem comes from esteemable acts. We can never feel good about ourselves if we don't feel good enough to pursue the things that are meaningful to us. Think about it, if we're afraid to make a change then that means we have no confidence in our abilities, and if that's the case then we will have a terrible self-image. The good news is even if we are afraid, we don't have to stay stuck there. As stated above, perhaps you don't have the technical skills or knowledge to pursue something new. That doesn't mean you cannot take steps to learn. The sooner you get honest with yourself about what you want and the sooner you are willing to take action toward it, the sooner you will feel better about yourself which will in turn begin the reclamation of your power and confidence.

I promise you that when you were a child and someone asked what you wanted to be when you grew up your answer was not: *"a sell-out, trading my soul for the almighty dollar"* or *"barely making ends meet in a mediocre job I hate."* When children are asked this question they answer with wonder, excitement, and a spark in their voice considering all the possibilities that await them. A note to the "realists," I get it, we cannot all be ballerinas. However, even if your dream was to be a dancer or a rockstar and that dream has faded out of reach, it doesn't mean that you cannot create a new dream grounded in your current reality. You can find a job that you are passionate about. The sooner you stop letting your fears and insecurities run the show the sooner you can start manifesting your ideal job.

If you're unhappy at work, then you're probably dealing with many of the challenges listed above. You do not have to continue this way. Pause. Be courageous. Take stock of your life and tell the truth to yourself about how deeply impacted you are by this untenable situation. Is it worth it to allow things to continue this way for another month, another year, or more? Tomorrow is a construct that we use to defer taking actions that scare us. You will never be "ready," the time is now. You deserve to be engaged in meaningful work that you enjoy where you are appreciated, respected, and compensated well for your contributions. And your friends and family deserve the best version of you that is filled up, available, and happy.

Judy Morris

The Only Thing We Have to Fear is Fear Itself

I never thought of myself as a fearful person. In fact, if you would have asked me what I was afraid of, I would have told you, nothing. Even as a child I didn't seem to experience the shyness or fear that's typical of someone that age. I was always confident about my ability to learn new skills, and was very comfortable communicating with adults, teachers, waiters, anyone. There was fearlessness and confidence within me. That confidence often made it difficult for me to connect with my own peers because they didn't feel comfortable in the situations, circumstances, or around the people where I felt most at home. Perhaps because they were afraid of becoming adults themselves. I couldn't understand why my friends wanted to remain young. To resist growing was incomprehensible to me. I couldn't wait to be an adult. I wanted that kind of power and freedom and understood that responsibility was the cost of admission. A small price to pay in my opinion. I couldn't fathom wanting to remain in a state of perpetual dependence upon authority figures. I wanted to be the authority figure in my own life.

The way I saw it, no matter how wonderful someone might have been, if I gave my power over to them, instead of retaining it myself, I would remain dependent on another person for my entire life. The more power we give over to others, the less we have over ourselves.

The thought of being independent, and responsible for my own life was my primary objective. I was ready to take on the world.

I never questioned what my career choice was going to be. Since I had been old enough to know what a career was, I knew that I wanted to be an attorney. It seemed a perfect fit, a position of great authority and responsibility.

However, that dream was never meant to be. My path took a different direction and I wound up on Wall Street instead. I enjoyed educating and counseling people about their finances. It was an exciting field, and it provided me with an opportunity to be the mistress of my own fate. I enjoyed massive success, and it was awesome.

However, as wonderful as my professional life was coming along, my personal life wasn't going well. As much as I loved everything that I was doing, underneath it all I was plagued with insecurity, and I was relying on alcohol to cope. You see, I didn't stay sober the first time. It took me 7 years and 3 separate attempts before I stayed sober. I was 3 years into my financial services career before I stopped drinking. I can't imagine how I would have studied for the series 7 sober.

What I didn't recognize at the time was that although I wasn't afraid of being responsible, the insecurity I was plagued by had everything to do with my own worthiness. I felt unworthy of the amazing opportunities coming my way. I felt unworthy of having a meaningful career and financial prosperity. I'll never forget the beautiful office setup I had after I was fully licensed, with my name and title etched on the glass: Judy Morris, Financial Advisor. As good as it felt, it still felt impossible at times. I had been so busy running away from my feelings of worthlessness and insecurity that I didn't even know they were there.

I dealt with my unworthiness with perfectionism. I set out to be the best financial advisor in the world. I was going to care about my clients more than anyone had ever cared. I was going to do everything right. My entire life became about proving my worth. I went to great lengths for my clients. Above and beyond. I became a workaholic.

I was afraid, terrified in fact that I was unlovable, unworthy of love. My biological father had rejected the idea that I was his daughter before I was even born, and his absence in my life was significant, it left an indelible mark on me. His rejection broke my heart.

In addition to my father's absence, I also interpreted my mother's personal turmoil and lack of relational skills as an indication of my worth. Looking back now, I can see clearly that she was desperately trying to create a stable home for us but at the time it seemed as though her attention was on everything and everyone else but me. We have very different personalities, and both needed very different things.

That being said, I was most hurt and upset with God. After all, didn't he set the whole thing up?

The way I saw it, God have given other little girls intact families, other daughters had fathers. Since he didn't give that to me, I must be worthless. He must have chosen me to incarnate as a perpetual Cinderella, slaving for everyone else yet never having anything of her own. Never to have a family or to be loved. The best I could hope for was a successful career and even that I was unsure of.

The truth of the matter was that the perfectionism and obsessive behaviors I thought made me so fabulous were all just a cover-up. I thought all my fervor was due to my commitment to excellence. When truth be told, it was a survival tactic to justify my value and earn my keep which worked great professionally. Not so great personally.

In romantic relationships, it's a whole different story. We can't act out in controlling or obsessive ways and expect things to go well. Being in a relationship with another person requires maturity, self-awareness, trust, the willingness to compromise at times as well as the ability to forgive and be forgiven.

I LOVED love and the idea of being in a relationship, at least the honeymoon stage of it. I was addicted to falling in love, the high dosages of oxytocin, and the unspoken promise of a bright future ahead. The intensity of the physicality of it, the person wanting to know all about me, being enchanted by me, paying so much attention to me. All of that was great. But as the saying goes, the honeymoon phase only lasts so long. Eventually, reality sets in and individual parties morph from being Prince Charming and Princess Wonderful to being two complex human beings with their own pasts, baggage, and maladaptive coping mechanisms that they created along the way to adapt and survive. That's the part where things get messy, and that's the part I couldn't deal with, inevitably ending my relationships.

You see I lacked the necessary ingredients to participate in a successful adult relationship. Not only was I incredibly emotionally immature, but I also lacked self-awareness, trust, and the ability and willingness to compromise. I also lacked the graciousness of forgiveness for myself and anyone else. I had a long road in front of me to uncover, dismantle, and reassemble my character.

I had built a character, my character, based on fear and driven by ego. A totally unsustainable dynamic if one wishes to have long-term meaningful relationships of any kind, let alone of the romantic variety.

Looking back, the reason that my relationships failed wasn't that the men didn't love me. It was because I wasn't clear about who I was, I wasn't being straight about want I wanted, and I lacked relational skills. I was playing the chameleon and when I couldn't keep that up anymore, I would create drama, blame them for my unhappiness and leave. I truly believe that those relationships were lessons along the way for both of us. I kept putting up my mask and kept attracting the match for the mask. Ultimately, each and every one of these relationships ran their course and proved themselves to be unsustainable.

Case in point, early in my sobriety, I was in a relationship with Theo. He was young, handsome, and came from a nice family. We were both sober and committed to that path. On paper, we looked great. However, I was still wearing a mask, and attracting matches based on that mask. I was presenting as a woman who wanted to have children, a woman open to adventure. Theo loved the outdoors, camping, and hiking. He loved children and had a successful career working with them. He couldn't wait to be a father. Theo was open, authentic, and clear about who he was and what he wanted. Deep down I knew that I didn't want children, but I was too afraid to admit it to myself because I thought it meant there was something wrong with me. I kept hoping that one day I would wake up and change my mind. That somehow, at a later date, and under the right circumstances, I would realize that motherhood was a role I desired. In addition, I dislike camping and hiking. I am very much, an indoor girl.

Theo and I had gotten engaged and were planning our wedding. I was set on getting married at the Ritz Carlton. I'll never forget taking him to the hotel. We walked into the lobby and while I was oohing and ahing, showing him everything, he told me that the whole place looked like an old ladies' parlor. Theo hated the hotel.

I was in disbelief. How was this even possible? How could he disdain luxury? It was then that I realized this was a charade I couldn't keep up. As much as I wanted to make it work with Theo, we were two very different people, who wanted very different things. In my sick head at the time, I thought that love meant he would abandon the things that he liked in favor of the things that I liked, which were, in my opinion, the right things because I had impeccable taste.

I moved from Theo to Arthur and became his Pygmalion. I was a modern-day Eliza Doolittle and Arthur was Professor Henry Higgins. Arthur and I met at a 12-Step meeting. I was speaking to the group, and he approached me with an excitement that I had never experienced before. Our connection wasn't indicative of sexual attraction, which was the only type of excitement I'd experienced from men, this was something more. It wasn't just that Arthur found me to be attractive physically, it was as though he could see my actual spirit and was excited about who I was as a person. Arthur was handsome and confident. He celebrated me and acknowledged my talents in ways that told me he was genuinely interested in getting to know me.

A group of us went to fellowship after the meeting and had a wonderful time chatting and trading stories. Arthur and I exchanged numbers afterward and our relationship began.

Although I've always had a history of dating men older than myself, Arthur was a little further outside my comfort zone, 24 years my senior. However, any reservations I thought I had about our age difference were put aside quickly. The pull to be with him was more powerful than any fears or insecurities I had. It was the strongest connection that I'd ever experienced with any other human being because it had transcended the physical realm - it was scary. Until then, I had never been with anyone who knew me better than I knew myself.

I had never been in a relationship with someone who saw through the façade of my ego, recognizing the real me and my untapped potential. I had never been with someone who was fully invested in my realizing my own potential. It was overwhelming at times.

Arthur was instrumental in my getting involved with personal development. Together, we attended an event about an upcoming transformational seminar. It wasn't an event I would've ever attended on my own, and had he not pressed me to register, I never would have signed up.

Attending that transformational seminar was one of the best decisions of my life as it put me steadily on a path to self-discovery that I would never have embarked on independently. Arthur's support, insistence, and even pressure, were the perfect combination to help push me beyond fears that I didn't even know I had. Allowing me the opportunity to create a future that I didn't know I wanted.

Perhaps it was his age, his wisdom, and his own personal experience that allowed Arthur to see everything so clearly. I don't know. However, what I do know is that he was an integral part of my journey. The most impactful mentor I have ever had. Artur's mentorship, unwavering belief in me, and determination for my success was a priceless gift that I didn't earn and definitely didn't deserve. But a gift that I am eternally grateful for.

As I'm sure you can imagine, being romantically involved with your mentor is sticky business. Being so raw and revealed romantically and psychologically to someone who is older, and more savvy is an imbalanced distribution of power. That imbalance put more of a burden on our relationship than it could withstand.

I was incredibly uncomfortable in my own skin to begin with but this level of focus this kind of intensity was too much for me. I wasn't capable of being a partner to him. I don't know if you can be a partner to someone who you're also being mentored by. I do know that it didn't work for us at that time and ultimately our relationship ended. I broke Arthur's heart and left him. Our romance was short-lived, but our friendship never died. His unwavering belief in me and his commitment to my success has always been in the background of our relationship.

I am deeply grateful to the 12 steps and the amends process which has enabled me to acknowledge my shortcomings, take responsibility for my part, and make amends to him. I am grateful for his mercy, his forgiveness, his continued friendship, and support. It's been an invaluable part of my journey.

Because I was still in the process of discovering myself, I continued looking for love and validation in all the wrong places. After my break-up with Arthur, I was in a very vulnerable place. I wasn't sure what was next for me. Then I met Samuel.

Samuel was different from other men. He was charming in a very subtle and disarming way. His kind eyes and jovial personality made him seem safe. We met at a party, and he liked me immediately making his intentions known to a mutual friend who eagerly played the part of our matchmaker.

Samuel was mesmerized by me, placing me on a pedestal that I never asked to be on. However, I was so desperate to be loved that I was willing to go to any length to get it. Including becoming whoever he needed me to be.

After being so revealed and raw in my relationship with Arthur, being in a relationship with someone who was so adoring without the same kinds of expectations was a welcome change.

I hadn't fully considered the consequences of jumping into another relationship before doing any real work to heal from the one that had just ended. I hadn't fully processed what had just happened. I was looking for relief, another form of escape.

The first six months of our relationship were a blissful honeymoon period. We were in a haze of oxytocin, drunk with dreams of the future. Things were going well in my career. I had just closed escrow on my first house, and we were moving into it together. Samuel was focused on his business and things seemed to be going his way. Everything was going well for us both, personally and professionally.

Then, out of the blue, I received a phone call from my brother who had been struggling with some challenges in life, asking if he might be able to live with me temporarily.

We had always been extremely close, and things were not working out for him at home. I can only imagine how difficult it must have been for him to be without a father. It isn't easy being a single mother to a teenage boy, just as it isn't easy being a teenage boy without a father.

My brother was 15 years old, the exact age I was when I left home. I was grateful that I was now in a stable and successful place in my career and relationship with a man who loved kids and had always wanted to be a dad. Samuel welcomed the opportunity to mentor my brother, and I wonder now, if he had thought it might be a good exercise, preparing us for the possibility of becoming parents in the future.

To be honest I was hesitant. As much as I loved my brother, I was at the pinnacle of success in my financial services career, and I was in the first year of a new relationship. I wasn't confident that it was a good idea but Samuel's insistence and reassurance that it was the right thing to do persuaded me to move forward.

My brother came to live with us, and I was able to provide him with opportunities he simply didn't have at home.

I had spent the last five years on my own personal development journey and had amassed tremendous resources and information I was able to share with him. I was able to provide my brother with access to personal development programs supporting his growth and my mentorship enabled him to overcome the challenges he was dealing with allowing him the opportunities to pursue his dreams of music and business.

My brother had always dreamt of being a professional musician and by the time he was 18 years old he was playing in a band, performing at shows, and had secured himself a position working with a boutique record label that represented some of his favorite bands.

It was a wonderful learning experience for him. As for me, it was an amazing opportunity to be able to contribute to my brother. I had always been conflicted about having children and being able to mentor him allowed me the experience of playing a parental role without having to commit to having a child. I am deeply grateful for that experience.

I loved being his big sister. It was a role that I never anticipated playing. My brother wasn't born until I was 14 years old and by that time, I didn't think I would ever have a sibling. I was reluctant to embrace the role at first but ultimately surrendered to it, and it has turned out to be one of the biggest gifts that God has ever given me.

Loving my brother cracked open my heart and made me look at myself deeper than I would have ever considered. Loving him committedly, and unconditionally, forced me to heal myself more deeply, and helped me become a better person. I would not be who I am in the world today had it not been for him and our relationship.

However, my commitment to my brother skewed my vision of my romantic relationship with Samuel. I was so busy trying to create the perfect family for us that I lost sight of creating the life that I wanted for myself. Samuel was very passionate about his dreams of being a husband and a father. He loved me deeply and wanted to create that life with me. Suddenly, I found myself in the middle of a scenario that I had never intended to manifest. We had essentially become parents 6 months into our relationship, and because we had never moved past the honeymoon phase as a couple, we never got to really know each other the way you do after that initial newness of a relationship wears off. Samuel wanted so badly to marry me, and I wanted so badly to provide a family for my brother, that we got engaged and then we got married. Once again, I found myself in the role of chameleon doing what I thought was right for everyone else but me.

That wedding day sticks out to me vividly because of the lack of joy in it. I felt utterly alone, isolated, and depressed. It felt more like I was producing an event for someone else's life; it didn't feel like mine.

Although I had done a fair amount of work on myself and had a certain level of self-awareness it was not sufficient to understand why what I was doing was a bad idea. Looking back now, I can recognize that it was a bad idea because I didn't want to marry Samuel and I didn't want to have children.

I was so sad on my wedding day. I had a facial scheduled that morning and when I laid down on the table, I started sobbing so violently that the esthetician was concerned. I think I scared her. She was begging me to stop crying, warning me that my face would be puffy, and it would ruin my pictures, but I couldn't stop.

My tears were the kind that came from my feet. They came from the depths of my soul. The tears felt endless, and I really couldn't connect the dots of where the pain was coming from. I can see clearly now that the pain related to my self-abandonment. The pain was in producing an event that had me committing my life to someone that I didn't want to be committed to. It was an event that was created for everyone else, except me.

I wanted to be a good example for the women I was sponsoring and mentoring, I wanted to be a good example for my brother. I was trying to be the person everyone else wanted me to be. I was totally disconnected from my own goals and dreams.

Samuel was a nice man, but he was not the man for me. I am confident that I would have discovered that had our relationship been allowed the chance to mature organically vs. being expedited as an instant family. I had been so disconnected from my intuition in an effort to please those around me, that I missed all the warning signs.

Samuel had an extremely enmeshed relationship with his father, who enabled him to pursue his artistic fantasies without any responsibility. Their relationship deeply interfered with our marriage, and I quickly discovered that I couldn't be in partnership with someone who already had a partner. Samuel made all of his decisions with his father, not with me. I didn't know anything about what was going on with his business until it went bankrupt. He had gotten involved in a project that became defunct because of a lack of preparation. He hadn't had a lawyer look at the agreement before he signed it and it wound up costing him the project and his business.

When I discovered what had happened, I was mortified. Samuel was someone who jumped headfirst into things he loved without doing the work to determine whether they were viable or not. The more I got to know him, the more clearly, I saw his utter lack of capacity to be honest with himself about his own limitations or the limitations of projects he wanted to pursue.

I was in the process of ending my career in finance which isn't something I anticipated doing. When I first began my career as a Financial Advisor at the ripe old age of 22 it never occurred to me that there would be anything else for me professionally. I felt that I had found my calling. I loved working with professionals, business owners, and families helping them to plan for their financial futures. Coaching was my natural habitat and providing financial coaching and investment guidance was my first entree to being paid for my advice. It was a perfect fit for many years. Then, in my mid 30's after having battled some of my own personal demons, I had changed. I was now on a road of spiritual growth and development, and spending my days discussing retirement plans, stock performance, and interest rates was no longer something that excited me.

Don't get me wrong, financial planning is important. It was just no longer what I wanted to focus on. I noticed that I started to lead my client conversations toward topics such as their health and well-being, work-life balance, and quality relationships. This was fine as an aside, but it being the focal point of our conversations was inappropriate. When reading *Psychology Today* took precedence over the *Wall Street Journal,* I knew I was in trouble. I realized that I needed to make a change and was terrified at the idea. I had spent the last 10 years building a profitable book of business and had a great reputation with countless referrals coming in every day. I didn't know what to do. How do you walk away from something that you know so well, and have worked so hard for?

Sometimes it takes an external crisis to foment a career transition. The banking and housing crisis was just that. I fell into a deep depression knowing that I was in no condition to steer my clients through this storm. It was no longer a question of my fears and concerns, it was now a matter of personal integrity. I was unwilling to put my clients at risk. I literally couldn't wait any longer, I had to make my move.

I met with my supervisor and transitioned my clients to the care of a highly qualified advisor and made my exit. My clients could not have been more understanding. Sure, they were sad to see me go. We had spent many years together creating financial success. But it was in their best interest as well as my own. Making a change like that takes courage, integrity, and faith in the process.

Now that Wall Street was behind me, I had to decide what the focus of my natural coaching expertise was going to be going forward. I had toyed with the idea of becoming a therapist. However, after a year in school, I realized that being a therapist wasn't the route I wanted to take. There were too many restrictions associated with that license that would have limited all the hands-on things I wanted to do with my future clients to help them heal. As a therapist, I wouldn't be able to drive a client to a 12-step meeting, help them with sorting out their meds with their doctors, or attending appointments with them. So, I decided that recovery coaching and case management were going to be the best option.

I had always been a skilled networker and collaborator, so it wasn't long before I was creating joint ventures with a few of my associates who were licensed therapists. Being a financial advisor is like being a financial case manager. When a client comes in you look at their entire picture. You determine if they need an accountant, an attorney, etc. and if so, you assemble the team and act as a liaison managing that team and holding the space for the big picture. This was a missing piece in the mental health world. Therapists were only able to spend 50 minutes per session with their patients and were not authorized to give direct advice. I had found a great niche and it was a powerful way to collaborate with mental health professionals while also supporting individuals who were about to embark on a journey I had already successfully traveled.

In addition to working as a recovery coach/case manager, I noticed that one of the recurring themes for my client conversations was their career. Looking back now, even when I was working with people on their finances, we would discuss their retirement, their income, and their career goals. As happens, once I made this discovery, the Universe presented me with an opportunity to partner with a local non-profit assisting their clients with employment preparation, and job readiness both in a one-on-one and group setting running their job clubs. I also had the opportunity to work as an employment specialist with individuals who were coming out of rehab, a mental health crisis, incarceration, or some other form or major life event.

I've had the privilege of working with people from all walks of life, from Google executives and entertainment personalities to entry-level customer service associates, administrative professionals, and bookkeepers. I've helped people to find traditional employment and supported others to start their own projects, businesses, and everything in between. With over 12 years' experience working with clients and empowering them to reach their goals, providing insight, support, and career resources for individuals who are committed to being fulfilled and on purpose in their work life, I still love the work I do. Every single day I get to help my clients design and live exceptional lives and careers. None of this would have been possible if I would have stayed in my comfort zone.

Clients often share with me that they are seeking "job security," and I tell them the same thing I'm going to tell you: There is no such thing as job security. Nothing is "secure" - life itself is risky. We get in our car and are taking a risk of being rear-ended. There's no way to prevent or control that from happening. It's the same idea when we get on a plane or attend an event. Every move we make involves risk. There is no way to avoid risk completely however we can reduce our exposure by employing risk management techniques.

I always recommend to my clients that we they're thinking about making a change, to not suppress the still small voice inside. Do the research, consider the options by working with an expert who's able to help you explore unchartered territory and assist you in mapping your course while providing support and guidance along the way. We don't have to travel our journey alone, nor should we. We're priceless, valuable, and worthy of all the abundance that we seek. We should never stop pursuing our goals and never give up on our dreams.

Of course, Samuel was very supportive of all of the changes I was making. He promised me the moon and stars. Promises that he couldn't keep even though he wanted to.

Samuel's immaturity, dishonesty, and financial irresponsibility pushed me further and further away until I ultimately ended our marriage. I will always be grateful to Samuel for the support he provided my brother was well as the love and kindness he always showed me.

Once again, I got to see how being a chameleon and abandoning myself simply didn't work because it is unsustainable. In the end, whoever it is we're pretending to be will never provide us with a truly fulfilling experience, and we'll have no choice but to revert to being ourselves, which will damage or destroy the relationships in which we're being chameleons.

I had become a cliché. I was a 35-year-old divorcee who was changing careers. I was afraid of being older and less attractive to men. I was afraid of ending up alone. I was afraid of failing in my new professional pursuits.

I was simply afraid.

I had sold my house, divorced my husband, and quit my job. I had completely shed my old identity, that of a successful Wall Street executive, the wife with an adoring husband. I was now standing in my truth in a way that I had never done before, and I was standing there alone.

That divorce launched me into two years of intensive healing and self-discovery. I had been diagnosed with PTSD very early in my sobriety, but I was not yet prepared to do anything about it at that time. I could not have delved deeply into my trauma when I was so newly sober. It was too much. I had to get some time under my belt, and I needed to have a solid program with a stable spiritual foundation before I was able to go there.

Now, I was finally willing and able to embark on this journey. This was my dark night of the soul. I had never been so uncertain, so insecure, or so aware of my own flaws and character defects.

I had finally come to the realization that the solution was not in finding another relationship or seeking security in a man or a company. This was next-level recovery work for me.

As terrifying as it all was, it was also incredibly transformational. I was able to dig into my own codependency and love addiction, discovering why I always needed to be in a relationship, and exploring the shadows behind my inability to be alone.

I started working with a Somatic Healer and dealing with my trauma. Let's take a moment to explore the subject of trauma.

Bessel van der Kolk, M.D., defines trauma as *"not the story of something that happened back then, but the current imprint of that pain, horror, and fear living inside [the individual]."* These events leave us stuck in a state of helplessness and terror, and result in a change in how we perceive danger. He goes on to say that: *"being traumatized means continuing to organize your life if the trauma were still going on unchanged and immutable as if every new encounter or event is constrained by the past."*

Trauma is often a topic of great misunderstanding. I cannot tell you how many times a client has assured me that they've never experienced any trauma because they relate to trauma as being physical violence, sexual abuse, or some other type of extraordinary external events. So often we presume that for an event or experience to qualify as being considered traumatic, it must be an act of God such as a planetary disaster, an earthquake, hurricane, a house burning down, or a parent being deployed and killed in a war.

I too was guilty of this. I was embarrassed by how the events of my childhood impacted me. I was not a survivor of incest, I hadn't experienced violent physical abuse, and so I thought that I should be happy and grateful for the life I had. It took a long time for me to recognize the nuances of my upbringing that negatively impacted me, the subtle things taking place like instability, neglect, and abandonment that impacted me so drastically. I had to have the courage to own my pain, examine it, and understand what it meant to me personally to know how best to deal with and ultimately heal it.

My favorite definition of trauma is any incident that occurs at a time when you feel extremely vulnerable and incapable of handling the situation. Said another way it's any situation that seems bigger than you, that you feel powerless over.

Trauma is exacerbated when it's happening to a small child who has not yet developed a sense of personality or any sense of their own power. Often children that have experienced trauma are diagnosed with complex PTSD because developmental trauma interferes with the development of our sense of self and sense of safety in the world. It also interferes with the development/regulation of our nervous system.

For example, let's say that you have a sibling who has special needs, and growing up, your family was constantly focusing their time and attention on that autistic sibling. Days and weeks were filled with doctor's appointments, and meetings with specialists, leaving your parents not only physically exhausted by the unexpected demands, but depleted financially because of the added medical bills, strain, and stress.

It's not something that happens intentionally any more than a hurricane destroying your home. A disabled sibling coming into the family was not an intentional trauma happening to you. But it is a trauma, nonetheless.

It was traumatizing because it took your parent's attention, affection, and even financial resources. It oftentimes left you alone in doctors waiting rooms or playing alone in your room while they were dealing with something bigger. Perhaps you didn't get to attend art classes or summer camp because of the financial drain on the family.

Perhaps being healthy and capable felt like a punishment because it seemed to rob you of the attention or affection that you longed to experience.

Or perhaps you had a parent that was suffering from substance abuse, a mental health issue, or a physical disability and they simply didn't have the emotional resources to expend on you. Maybe your parent had a physical disability such as MS or were diagnosed with cancer. The trauma of having someone so seriously ill in the house, along with all the sadness, fear, and uncertainty associated with the illness, turned the focus onto the sick person and off of everyone else.

Perhaps your mother was an incest survivor and every time you tried to dress up, put on make-up or a short skirt you were accused of being a bad girl. She turned your curiosity and interest in boys into a crime, a bad behavior, a warning that were preparing for life as a prostitute seeking her next John.

Perhaps she berated you about how your body was disgusting and dirty, how you needed to hide it, be ashamed of it, afraid of it. Perhaps she projected her own unhealthy fears, insecurities, and unresolved issues onto you. Issues you then internalized and allowed to tarnish the way you felt and saw your body, leaving you feeling ashamed and dirty even though no one had ever touched you.

A holistic approach to trauma defines trauma not as an event, but rather as a disruption and overwhelm to our body-mind's capacity to adapt and thrive. Trauma can occur when there is too much too soon, too much for too long, not enough for too long, a person's power and agency having been taken away from them, stressors outweighing the resources available to navigate them, anytime our primal protective instincts, intuitions, and responses are thwarted, or when there is not enough time, space, or permission to heal or grieve our losses.

We must also consider social, developmental, and cultural factors when reflecting on trauma. By not acknowledging these contextual factors our examination will remain incomplete.

Symptoms of trauma may occur immediately or emerge over time from the compounding stress and challenges of processing and adapting to the experiences of life. These symptoms may emerge as the body and mind attempt to cope with and resolve stressors. Their effects may include physical symptoms such as headaches, dizziness, tightness in the body, muscle tension, digestion challenges, and constrictions around the breath.

Emotional symptoms such as depression, disinterest in activities, an inability to feel, fear, anxiety, panic, overwhelm, loss of choice, difficulty feeling comforted, anger, and shame.

Psychological symptoms may include presentations such as dissociation, mental rumination, low self-worth, negative self-talk, self-blame, and memory challenges.

Trauma can also impact the ability to connect relationally or socially resulting in isolation, loneliness, and attachment disorders, leading to feelings of powerlessness, helplessness, and groundlessness. It can interfere with one's ability to feel real in body and mind, disrupting our very sense of existence, and taking us away from the present moment. However, as noted by Dr. Peter Levine, *"Trauma is a fact of life. It does not have to be a life sentence."* The courage to acknowledge symptoms is the first step to healing trauma.

If you are feeling unworthy, unloved, punished, afraid, uncomfortable, or any of the other effects above, it's always worth exploring further. You are not crazy. I can guarantee you that by tracing those effects and feelings back to their origin, you'll find something that took place in your childhood that was either covert, or unclear. It may be something as simple as your father getting promoted and your family having to move, leaving your best friend, which was the worst thing that you could have imagined happening at the time, and an experience that you never got over. Who knows how things affect us, we are all unique individuals, and we deserve the love and attention to explore the way that things impact us?

Dis-ease whether it is presenting as discomfort, anxiety, chronic fatigue, or fibromyalgia is an indicator of something that isn't right, and we deserve to explore to find out what the root issue is, and how it's impacting us so that we have an opportunity to heal. As Bessel Vander Kolk says, "the body keeps the score," our bodies house within them, memories, and reactions to events from the past not only in our own lives but in the lives of our ancestors.

There might be things troubling us that aren't even ours. We all incarnate with seven generations of trauma that are impacting us in some form or fashion, depending on our culture, as well as our family line.

Let's take a look at transgenerational trauma which can be defined as a collective experience that affects groups of individuals who share a cultural identity, ethnicity, nationality, or religious belief. It can also be applied to single families or individual parent-child dyads. Also referred to as intergenerational trauma, this phenomenon can be found in situations where the descendants of a single person or cultural group who experiences a terrifying event, go on to show adverse emotional and behavioral reactions to event that are similar in their own lives. Specific reactions vary by generation but can include shame, increased anxiety, guilt, a heightened sense of vulnerability, helplessness, low self-esteem, depression, suicidality, substance abuse, and difficulty in relationships with others.

I'm a big believer in the concept of having a treatment team. Healing is not an independent endeavor. After all the first word in the first step is: WE.

I personally participated in talk therapy, which was incredibly supportive, informative, and healing, I also worked a strong 12-step program, and even ventured into working the steps in another 12-step fellowship. I participated in transformational seminars and workshops of various kinds. I experimented with acupuncture and reiki healing. I was no stranger to treatment modalities, but when I decided to explore PTSD treatments, I learned about somatic healing which was something that was new to me.

Inspired to study stress on the animal nervous system, Dr. Peter Levine, founder of Somatic Experiencing, recognized that while animals live constantly under threat of death, they show no symptoms of trauma. He discovered that trauma is a result of the third survival response to perceived life threat, which is freeze. When fight and flight are not options, we freeze and immobilize, like "playing dead," and making us less of a target. However, because this reaction is time-sensitive and involves the releasing or discharging of the energy prepared for a fight or flight response, when we are unable to complete the immobility or freeze response, that energy charge stays trapped within the body. Thus, communicating to ourselves that we are still under threat.

I discovered that somatic trauma therapy offered techniques to help individuals sense and regulate their own physiology and states of being. This includes developing additional internal and external resources, building trusting and co-regulatory relationships, learning to turn inward with compassion, being invited deeper into the body, and being given time and space to process the trauma. These somatic techniques unwind trauma and restore well-being. Benefits include restoring the body as a place of safety while helping to expand the capacity to process body (preverbal and nonverbal) memory, metabolizing unprocessed emotions, completing thwarted (incomplete) stress responses, and restoring our optimal relationship to ourselves and the world around us.

Because of the foundational spiritual work and healing I had already completed, I was capable and available to receive this new, higher level of healing. It was scary at times, to feel such big unprocessed feelings emerge from in my body. There was a lot of crying, a lot of respiratory reactions, and a lot of writing. But at the end of it all, I have never been freer. The only thing I had to fear was fear itself. It took a lot of failed relationships including two divorces before I developed the courage and willingness to really look at myself and face my fears. Only by facing my fears and telling the truth could I ever be me. And only by being me and developing relational skills could I ever hope to successfully participate in a long-term committed partnership.

Being sober and doing the work in my alcohol recovery program wasn't sufficient to heal all the other stuff. The journey never ends. Recovery and self-discovery are ongoing processes. Especially for someone with complex developmental trauma. However, I am here to tell you that it is possible, and worth every moment.

Judy Morris

A New Pair of Glasses

It wasn't until I started working on myself that I discovered how playing the victim is rooted in self-pity, and self-pity is rooted in self-centered fear.

Webster's dictionary defines a victim as someone who is subjected to oppression, hardship, or mistreatment. And although I had certainly experienced times of hardship, mistreatment, and oppression, those times were behind me, and I didn't need to continue living in a perpetual reaction to those times. The definition of self-pity is a self-indulgent dwelling on one's own sorrows or misfortunes. OUCH! That hit the nail on the head for me. I had been dwelling on my sorrows and misfortunes, focusing on them, ruminating about them, drinking over them, causing drama with men over them, and sabotaging my future because of them. In fact, when I looked back over my life, I had successfully removed myself from unfavorable circumstances at the age of 15. So, what was I still so upset about? It was as if my life were a record and there was a scratch that kept the same few chords repeating over and over again.

All my life I had felt victimized by my circumstances. I thought that I was eternally doomed to be depressed. I thought that I was broken, unlovable, and all alone in the world. I thought that because I had incarnated into what I believed to be unfavorable, unchangeable circumstances, there was no hope for me. It wasn't until I got sober and started working a program of recovery that a little glimmer of hope crept in, that I began to wonder if maybe healing was possible. Because I had felt so victimized by my circumstances, I thought I was destined to remain a victim. I didn't know yet that while I was powerless over my circumstances — it didn't mean that I was powerless over who I was going to be in the face of those circumstances. I didn't know that the truth of the matter was I wasn't suffering over what had happened to me as much as I was suffering over what I had made it mean. I had made it mean that I was unlovable, that I wasn't worthy, that I had been forsaken by my Higher Power.

I didn't start therapy until I was 25 years old, and even then, it was only because I'd tried staying sober twice before with no success. I was afraid of relapsing, and I knew I needed help. The first few therapists I met with were not a match. However, I didn't give up. I kept searching, knowing I would find the right person and I did. He was a brilliant, patient, experienced, and talented psychotherapist.

I can still remember our very first session. After all the "suffering" and struggling I had been experiencing, in a single session he laid out my problem. I didn't like what he said. I didn't want to return. However, there was a little voice inside of me that said: "You trust him, you paid him, why not listen to him? Why not try to see this from his perspective?"

Here's the funny thing, my therapist was not a member of a 12-step fellowship, in fact, he knew very little about such programs, so he certainly was not quoting their material, and yet, what he said was exactly the same thing being discussed in the meetings I attended, and the literature that outlined the theory extensively. At the end of our session, after he had listened to me for 50 minutes, he told me very simply, the same thing that the big book had been telling me however, I hadn't been willing to hear it. My therapist pointed out that I was completely self-centered, that I really didn't want to stop drinking, and that I actually didn't care about anyone other than myself.

The big book says: "Selfishness - self-centeredness! That, we think, is the root of our troubles. Driven by a hundred forms of fear, self-delusion, self-seeking, and self-pity, we step on the toes of our fellows, and they retaliate. Sometimes they hurt us, seemingly without provocation, but we invariably find that at some time in the past we have made decisions based on self which later placed us in a position to be hurt. So, our troubles, we think, are basically of our own making."

You see, I was masterful at getting people to feel sorry for me. All the therapists I had met with before were feeding into my story of self-pity. No wonder I didn't resonate with them. This person was different. He wasn't afraid of me or my pain. He refused to believe that my pain was bigger than me or that I couldn't transcend it. Here was a person who wanted more for me. Who knew that if I didn't grow up and take responsibility for my life, I would never be able to stay sober.

By the way, that was the turning point. After meeting with this therapist, I NEVER drank again. My work with him combined with the work I was doing within the 12-step program really helped me excavate all the dis-ease in my mind and heart, allowing me the space I needed to finally begin to heal.

Those first two years we dove deep into my mind, uncovering all of the inaccurate, self-destructive, interpretations I had created in reaction to my upbringing. We looked at my life. All the baggage within my family, the stuff that happened growing up and in my relationships. My therapist helped me see my thoughts as thoughts and not as the truth. He helped me to recognize them as just one set of interpretations. He supported me in seeing that although I didn't get to pick the hand I was dealt, I had a choice as to how I was going to play that hand. He encouraged me to take a closer look at my many relationship dances and taught me how to learn new ones.

Please note that I'm not in any way setting out to minimize my own or anyone else's trauma. What I am seeking to do is illustrate that although situations or experiences may have been bigger than us at the time they occurred, we don't have to allow them to stay that way. Therapists and healers can go with us to the scary places we previously had to navigate alone, guiding us toward taking back our power. I'm here to witness to you that I have done it. And believe it or not, the process was nowhere near as hard as I thought it was going to be and yet, in some ways it was harder. But hands down, it was worth it.

Through the work I was doing on myself I discovered that all my fear of failure, anxiety, repetitive negative thoughts, and fear of nothing changing was an automatic response to the negative attitude I had developed in reaction to unfavorable and oftentimes traumatic circumstances.

I didn't know what to do with all of that until I got into recovery. The first prayer I learned was the serenity prayer which states: *"God grant me the serenity to accept the things I cannot change; Courage to change the things I can; And wisdom to know the difference."*

I learned once again that although I couldn't change what happened, I could change my relationship with it. I could change my attitude about it.

No, I still didn't know my biological father. No, he didn't fight for me or to play a part in my life. I have no idea why he made that choice. But I do know for a fact that it has NOTHING to do with my worth. I realized that I didn't need to continue to interpret his rejection and abandonment as such.

Yes, my grandparents moved out of state and left me behind. Yes, it seemed like the end of the world at the time. Yes, it was traumatizing and terrifying. Yes, it was bigger than I was at 12 years old. But I wasn't 12 years old anymore. I was no longer powerless over my environment. Their decision to move didn't affirm my unworthiness of a safe and loving home. Their plans didn't have to mean that I was unlovable. I no longer needed

to continue to fuel the fire that was that story that was fueling my
alcoholism.

*"And acceptance is the answer to all my problems today. When I am
disturbed, it is because I find some person, place, thing, or situation—
some fact of my life—unacceptable to me, and I can find no serenity until
I accept that person, place, thing, or situation as being exactly the way it is
supposed to be at this moment. Nothing, absolutely nothing, happens in
God's world by mistake. Until I could accept my alcoholism, I could not stay
sober; unless I accept life completely on life's terms, I cannot be happy. I
need to concentrate not so much on what needs to be changed in the
world as on what needs to be changed in me and in my attitudes."*
  - Alcoholics Anonymous: The Big Book

It's common for people who've experienced traumatic childhoods to
seek out a "savior," someone to rescue them from all of their sadness and
fear, providing a utopia for them. That was certainly my fantasy. However,
as I sought help, I came to the realization that no one was coming. There
was no one out there. There was no man or career that was going to
rescue me from myself. I am now and will always be, the one that I have
been waiting for. I had to grow up and stop hurting myself. It was an inside
job that I needed to handle myself.

This was an incredible revelation. I had known these things on a
surface level because so many recovery and transformational personal
development programs talk about the subject, they all speak in depth
about the importance of personal responsibility. But knowing something
and living something are two very different things. As much as I
understood intellectually the concept of independence and self-
responsibility subconsciously, I had still been pursuing relationships with

men or career success to alleviate my fears, insecurities, and feelings of unworthiness.

Coming into my own as an independent, sovereign woman who no longer sought outside circumstances to fix her has been a triumph. I had wanted so desperately, for so long, to be that kind of woman, and the journey was long and arduous. There were countless layers of ego to discover and discard, ancestral trauma to work through, generations of codependency, martyrdom, and self-abandonment.

On the other side of it all was a brand-new view of myself and the world. I was finally able to put everything in perspective. I was able to forgive myself and others on a deeper level.

I was able to give up the need to belong to anything outside of myself. I had finally come to a place of belonging – belonging to myself - belonging to my Higher Power - and that was enough for me.

So how did I get that change of perspective? I did the work. And although it is an inside job, it's not work that can be done alone. Think of it like climbing Mount Everest. There are Tibetan people called Sherpas living on the high southern slopes of the Himalayas in eastern Nepal who provide support for foreign trekkers and mountain climbers.

I needed Sherpas not saviors. BIG difference. Ultimately this is what therapists, healers, sponsors, and mentors are, they're spiritual, psychological, emotional, energetic sherpas, people who know the terrain, have navigated it successfully, and now help others to do the same.

Once I had gone through the first round of healing, once I had completed the 12-steps, I knew that I had to show others the way. There's a saying in the rooms that I found to be very true: "you have to give it away to keep it."

There's no mistake that the 12th step is about carrying a message and practicing the principles. I must put what I have learned into practice and be willing and available to help others do the same. That doesn't mean I have to quit my job and become a full-time coach or healer (although that does happen to some of us), however, I do need to give some of my time to the task of helping others. I found that my healing process was not complete until I started sharing the message with others.

The first 18 months of my sobriety were fine. I went to meetings; I worked the steps with a sponsor. I took commitments and participated. I did all the things that had been suggested of me but there was still something missing. I had made some progress and was feeling better, but I was still depressed and felt very much alone. So, I decided to do something different. I decided to go to a meeting held on the other side of town, one that I had never attended before, in hopes of mixing things up and meeting new people. That's where the magic happened for me. It just so happened that the group I visit was my tribe. I connected with people right away.

The first night I was invited by multiple people to speak at other meetings. The following week I was asked to sponsor someone. Although I had been sober for over 18 months, I had never been asked to sponsor anyone before. I was honored and excited. I LOVED the message of the program, and I couldn't wait to share that message with another woman. Every night of the week I had something lined-up, meeting at a coffee shop before the meeting to go through the book or work a step, during the days sometimes taking an outreach call.
I had held very high-level positions in my career and had achieved professional success in a variety of ways, I had worked on myself and participated in therapy, and worked the steps myself. But I must say that there was something magical in sharing this message with someone else.

Working with a newcomer gave me a sense of purpose, direction, and meaning that I had only ever experienced when mentoring my brother.

There's a magic in service that cannot be overestimated. Service is about giving without expectation of receiving anything in return. It is not an ego-driven pursuit. We give freely.

One of my favorite quotes of all time is by George Bernard Shaw:

"This is the true joy in life: being used for a purpose recognized by yourself as a mighty one, being a force of nature instead of a feverish, selfish little clod of ailments and grievances, complaining that the world will not devote itself to making you happy. I am of the opinion that my life belongs to the whole community and as long as I live, it is my privilege to do for it what I can. It is a sort of splendid torch which I have got hold of for the moment and I want to make it burn as brightly as possible before handing it on to future generations."

Healing isn't personal. When we go through the healing process, we have a unique and sacred opportunity to help heal our family line. We have the chance to heal our ancestors who may not have had the opportunity, education, or resources to do the work for themselves. In addition, we clear the line in front of us, breaking the cycle and becoming the heroes or heroines of our family's story.

In addition, we're able to impact our community. We don't have to be a therapist, coach, or healer to impact others. Marianne Williamson writes about this concept beautifully in her book, *"A Return to Love."*

"Our deepest fear is not that we are inadequate. Our deepest fear is that we are powerful beyond measure. It is our light, not our darkness that most frightens us. We ask ourselves, who am I to be brilliant, gorgeous, talented, and fabulous? Actually, who are you not to be? You are a child of God. Your playing small does not serve the world. There is nothing

enlightened about shrinking so that other people will not feel insecure around you. We are all meant to shine, as children do. We were born to make manifest the glory of God that is within us. It is not just in some of us; it is in everyone and as we let our own light shine, we unconsciously give others permission to do the same. As we are liberated from our own fear, our presence automatically liberates others."

All it takes to kindle the fire of desire in someone else is to be an example.

How many of us have seen someone get a new job, lose weight, tone up, save money, or clear their credit score? We see their results and become inspired, wanting to know what they've done because we want some of that magic too. We all have that ability to influence, inspire, and impact others just by being an example to our friends, neighbors, and coworkers.

The way we communicate may be the only way that person is able to hear the message that we're carrying. When we share our story with someone in a way that they're able to hear and comprehend, we inspire them to take action and heal themselves.

Not to mention, by "giving it away," by sharing our message, whatever that message may be, we get to deepen our own relationship to it, our own understanding of it, strengthening our own resolve and conviction.

As I've shared throughout this book, I struggled with self-love, self-esteem, and my attitude. The answer for me, was to get out of self. It was to have my life be about something bigger than myself. By committing my life to be of service, to sharing, to being a contributing member of society, I have in turn learned how to love myself, and heal the part of me that felt broken and alone for so many years. We cannot be broken or alone if we're empowering others. It isn't possible. We cannot dwell in darkness if we are sharing our light with others.

Included here's a letter I wrote regarding my experience of mentoring women and how being of service has positively impacted my life. I share it here in hopes of inspiring you on your own journey of service.

To My Girls:

My beautiful girls, how I've loved you, how I've longed to help you heal and find love. I loved you when I didn't know how to love myself. I learned about your challenges and committed to find solutions.

In the beginning I thought it was about me helping you. I see now, that in loving you, I've learned to love myself, and therefore, I am the one who has been healed.

You have been my mirror. I have seen the depths of despair in you - but also, infinite hope. I have looked at some of you, and been horrified at what I found there, reflected. The darkest parts of my own self, that I had not yet considered accepting, had me judge, condemn, and reject more than a few of you. In addition, the darkest parts of myself that you had yet to recognize, accept, or acknowledge in yourselves, caused more than a few of you to outright reject me. Those were the most painful moments, but I used them to fuel my own transformation. Those were moments that made me dig deep into the recesses of my own inauthenticity, and inspired courage beyond limitation, which has in turn, made me a better human being.

In the depths of my love for you I encountered my utter inadequacy to the task. How could this self-centered, self-seeking, insecure, judgmental alcoholic ever love you? Rather than be dissuaded, I became obsessed with removing any barriers that seemed to separate us. My love for you, has been a beacon of light, that has guided me to a rich and profound spiritual awakening. You have taught me how to serve, how to contribute, and how to give.

The greatest achievement in my life has been participating in your journey. I see my imprint woven into the fabric of your recovery, I hear it in your speech, and see it in your life. I remember the moments when I had the honor of teaching you these lessons. Now, seeing you live them, is the grandest award beyond any material success. I am a rich woman, grossly overpaid.

The intimacy, connection, and healing that we have shared have been the most precious moments in my life. Nothing brings me more happiness than contributing to you.

I have learned that all the love I had been seeking "out there" was an illusion. I am love. Love is an infinite resource, and an inexhaustible well that lives and grows inside of me. When I contribute that to you, it always returns to me, multiplied abundantly!

Now that we've addressed the power of service and sharing, let's talk about the power of gratitude.

I've learned to be grateful for all of it. For everything that's happened because all of it has shaped me to be the woman I am today, and I love who I am today.

When we make a conscious habit to express appreciation for our lives, instead of expressing disdain for what we don't have, and resentment about everything that's happened to us in the past, the Universe listens and responds with even more love.

Life is perfectly imperfect. Sometimes things happen and we react negatively. That's normal. However, what we want to focus on here is how we can shift our autopilot default setting from seeing the glass as half empty to seeing it as half full.

An attitude of gratitude forces us to go beyond the minutia of the day-to-day and focus instead on the bigger picture. In turn, we're better able to bounce forward when challenges occur in life.

An attitude of gratitude has us operating from a place of abundance instead of a place of scarcity and fear. No matter what we're facing, we always have a choice as to what we focus on.

People who are grateful give thanks for everything in their lives, not just when things are going their way. They find things to be grateful for even in the face of challenges because they know that gratitude is an attitude that must be cultivated and nurtured in order to be maintained. While it can take time and continued effort to make this shift, it's more than worth it! What we focus on increases and when we focus on what we don't have, we never have enough. Conversely, when we focus on what we are grateful for, then we always have more than what we need.

In order to turn an attitude of gratitude into a sustainable habit, our foundation for feelings of gratitude cannot be dependent on our circumstances.

So, even on the days when it feels like nothing is going right, especially on those days, it's imperative that we make the effort to find a silver lining and give thanks for what is working.

Gratitude isn't just a good idea because it feels better, it improves our mental health. Psychologists have found that negative events have a greater impact on our brains than positive ones, they refer to this as the negative bias. And it only takes a moment to give thanks for what we have, instead of complaining about what we don't.

Here are a few practices that can help to develop this invaluable perspective:

- **Keep a gratitude journal**

How many times throughout the day do we experience things that we should be grateful for, only to forget about them the next day. That is why keeping a journal of what we're grateful for is a good idea. By doing so we're not only rewiring our brain to focus on the good but keeping track of positive memories that we can go back and reflect on, giving us a much-needed boost on a challenging day.

As with developing any new habit, consistency is key. Make sure to create a routine of writing in your journal daily. I recommend choosing a specific time of day. For example, I like to write mine at night. I sit back and reflect upon everything that happened throughout the day and express my gratitude for it. It's a beautiful thing to fall asleep with a grateful heart.

- **Communicate your gratitude**

Sharing our gratitude with others helps us to expedite this change in attitude. I encourage you to acknowledge others for the ways that they have impacted you and your gratitude for it. What we put out comes back to us multiplied abundantly. The more we express our love and gratitude for others the more present we'll be for all of the good and love in our lives which help us to feel more connected with others. Listen to the promptings in your spirit. Send that bouquet of flowers, drop that "thinking of you" card in the mail, send a friend a copy of a book you're enjoying for no other reason than to share.

- **Celebrate your wins big or small**

I don't know where you live, but here in Los Angeles, home of the Academy Awards, The Golden Globes, and the Grammys, I was taught to focus on the big wins and to forget about the smaller ones. However, I've found that this is a mistake. By paying attention only to big wins, we miss the opportunity to celebrate all of our successes along the way. In fact, if we only counting the Academy Awards in our life, we can quickly become defeated and uninspired.

Remember, life is an experience, not an achievement. When who we are is not defined by the end goal but rather, by the person e become along the way, life is a much more satisfying experience.

Slow your pace, take time to pause, and savor the little things. Instead of stressing yourself out by obsessing about the future or dwelling on the past, you can practice the art of being present in the moment. After all, this is it, this moment is all any of us has. Enjoy it.

- **Meditate**

Meditation is a powerful practice in self-awareness. The goal isn't to silence our thoughts but rather, to become an active observer of them. The process of meditation is all about allowing the mind to do what it does and accept it as it is. Not every thought needs to be believed or acted upon. Mediation can create the much-needed distance to provide objectivity.

If you're someone who struggles with mediation, do not be discouraged. I highly recommend starting with a short 5–10-minute guided mediation. And, since we are on the topic of gratitude, you can find a variety of mediations focused on gratitude available to stream on YouTube. Start there.

Science shows that meditation can help build areas of our brain and rewire it to enhance positive traits such as focus, and decision making, while diminishing the less positive traits including fear and stress

When we master the mind, we master our emotions. Suddenly, we start to experience flow instead of chaos. There is more ease. Reactivity reduces, and our ability to handle life's challenges gracefully increases. No matter what our age or circumstance, it's never too late to start cultivating an attitude of gratitude.

Think about what you're grateful for? Give thanks for what you have, the food on your table, the roof over your head. Whatever you can think of. Do this every day for 30 days and watch your life change. Gratitude truly has the power to transform our lives from mediocre to miraculous!

Experts in the medical and scientific fields continue to find evidence that our thoughts — positive and negative — don't just have psychological effects, they also have physical effects on our bodies.

It's easy to assume that a disease or illness is the source of our fatigue or chronic pain, but have you ever considered that negative thinking could also be the reason? Pessimism affects more than just our mood. In fact, doctors have found that people who are highly negative are more likely to suffer from degenerative brain diseases, cardiovascular problems, and digestive issues, as well as experiencing prolonged recovery from sickness at slower rates than those with a positive mindset. Negative thoughts and emotions are a natural response to tragedy or disaster. But prolonged negativity can result in serious health problems. Negativity catapults our bodies into stress and 'fight-or-flight' mode. Our bodies are designed to deal with stressful situations by releasing cortisol into the bloodstream, which makes us more alert and focused. Though some stress is good for us, too much can be detrimental to our health. Extended periods of negativity slow digestion and decrease our immune system's ability to fight inflammation. This is one reason why negative people are more likely to get sick than optimists.

The advantages of positive thinking are not to be discounted or ignored, they include reduced stress, better overall physical and emotional health, longer life span, and better coping skills.

In addition, a positive self-image is a key to living a happy and healthy life. Research shows that people who feel confidently about themselves are more adept at problem-solving, better decision-makers, more comfortable taking calculated risks, more confident in asserting themselves, and strive to achieve their personal goals. There's an entire field of study devoted to what's now known as Positive Psychology. Further reason to invest in the development of positive thinking, and optimal mental health.

I want to expand on the topic of positive thinking. Solution-oriented thinking is directly connected to positive thinking. If we're dwelling on negativity than the way we relate to a problem will also be negative. If we're approaching something from the position of being a victim, the solution will be difficult to find as we'll view the problem as evidence of our victim circumstance. Victims are disempowered by problems because they seem unresolvable. Let's face it, if we're not empowered, everything seems unresolvable.

When we focus on the solution, instead of the problem, we're coming from a positive perspective. Solution-oriented thinking comes from being empowered and it allows us to see whatever challenge we're facing as an opportunity to learn something, resolve something, or make a change.

So far, we've looked at the cost of playing the victim and wallowing in self-pity, we've talked about the power of having a positive attitude and taking our focus off the past, accepting the things that we cannot change, switching our focus to reframing our relationship to the past, and creating an empowered attitude around it. We've talked about the power of positive/solution-oriented thinking, personal responsibility, and service. Now, we're going to deepen the conversation by looking at how our relationships impact our attitudes and beliefs.

Motivational speaker Jim Rohn famously said that *"we are the average of the five people we spend the most time with."*

This relates to the law of averages, which is the theory that the result of any given situation will be the average of all outcomes. Salespeople, entrepreneurs, and other successful individuals know that in order to increase their wins, they've also got to increase their losses.

When it comes to relationships, we're greatly influenced — whether we like it or not — by those closest to us. They affect our way of thinking, our self-esteem, and our decisions. Of course, we're each our own person, but research has shown that we're more affected by our environments than we think.

While it's ideal to be closely surrounded by positive, supportive people who want us to succeed, it's also necessary to have critics. According to a study in the Journal of Consumer Research, experts seek and respond to negative feedback to make progress and improve, while novices prefer receiving only positive feedback.

The more successful we become, the more criticism we face. Glenn Llopis shared in Forbes magazine that there are 6 types of people who help to build our mental toughness, including doubters, critics, and the envious, because without them, we'd never sharpen our skills or develop a tough enough skin to take the big risks that deliver even bigger rewards.

Judy Morris

Boundaries

"People learn how to treat you based on what you allow and accept from them, and others." – Amanda E. White

What is a boundary? A boundary is a limit that defines us in our relationship to someone or something. Boundaries can be physical and tangible, or emotional and intangible.

Boundaries are to people what traffic laws are to the road. They provide clear expectations of how we should behave on our relationship road, with clear consequences for breaking the rules, and protecting all parties involved, or on the road.

Most of the women I work with say that they'd like to stand up for themselves, say no, and honor their values, limits, and boundaries without feeling guilty. And yet, they cannot seem to do it. Too often, they sell themselves out for the approval of others rather than to risk losing favor with someone, even temporarily. Why are we so concerned with others over ourselves? Why are women so filled with guilt?

Consider that we may feel guilty not because we've done anything wrong but instead, because we're confused. We haven't distinguished the difference between what we're responsible for and what we're not. We haven't yet established where our boundaries lie.

Contrary to popular belief, we are NOT responsible for anyone's feelings. When I say anyone, that includes our children, spouse, parents, etc. In fact, we are powerless over other people's reactions.

We feel guilty because our action or lack of action failed to meet the expectation of another.

We feel guilty because we think that being a good mom, wife, daughter, etc. loving our family means they are happy all the time or not "mad" at us. We feel guilty at work because we see others working 80 hours per week without complaining, or asking for time off, so we think we should mirror those same behaviors. We're trapped in a comparison game, comparing our needs and desires with others, as well as looking outside of ourselves for approval, for wholeness. We're looking outside of ourselves because we were never taught to look inside. Perhaps even more to the point, we cannot honor our boundaries if we don't have any.

"The soul's integrity is the one and only thing that matters. We have no problem but to bring this about, no need but to obtain this; for having this, we have all…No sacrifice can be too great to ensure the integrity of one's soul. Anything, anything that stands in the way of that must be given up. Cost what it will involve what it may, the integrity of the soul must be preserved; for ALL other things conduct, health, prosperity; for ALL other things as, health, prosperity, life itself – follow upon that…It matters not what the thing may be that is standing between us and our true contact with our Higher Power. It must go. For what will it profit a man if he gains the whole world and forfeits his soul?"

- Emmet Fox

If we think that there's anything that will bring us happiness other than our own wholeness, we're sadly mistaken. The only path to true happiness is wholeness and we cannot be whole if the integrity of our soul is broken. Anyone who has participated in a 12-step program knows that we do not concern ourselves with goals and dreams at the beginning. We began by restoring integrity, completing the past, and becoming whole. Once this task has been completed, even in its most basic form, we have moved out of fear, into faith, and from there we stand on solid ground with the ability to create an inspiring future.

Judy Morris

There's No Place Like Home

The Wizard of Oz is an excellent cinematic example of codependency. Here we have a character named Dorothy who desires to go beyond the little farm she lives on, to explore the world and pursue her dreams. However, she struggles with fear and insecurity to take such a bold, risky, action. It's a terrifying thought for a young woman in 1939 (the year that film was released), to leave her family, her home, and the only life she's ever known. Dorothy ends up exploring her fantasy in a dream after a tornado descends upon her home, causing her to fall, hit her head, and doze into a deep slumber. The film then takes us into Dorothy's dreams, where we accompany her on a journey toward a place called the Emerald City, in a land called Oz.

We get to witness as she navigates the confusion of her own insecurities as well as the self-doubt she confronts in this new and unfamiliar world. And, when all is said and done, she does remarkably well. After all the obstacles, challenges, and ultimate triumphs she experiences in her dream, Dorothy awakens from her slumber, terrified of what she had just experienced only to abandon her deepest desires, to leave Kansas, and condemns herself to a life of mediocrity on her family's farm.

It's no wonder that the only outlet for Dorothy's fantasy was in her dream. Dreams are often the place where our suppressed desires or other unresolved issues reside. They come up from our subconscious during our sleep to process and play themselves out in fascinating and unexpected ways.

So why do people abandon themselves, their dreams, and their deepest desires to instead hold on to something that's familiar and safe but unfulfilling?

Fear. Fear of failure, fear of being alone, fear of being rejected, fear of being wrong, all different forms of fear.

"...fear. This short word somehow touches about every aspect of our lives. It was an evil and corroding thread; the fabric of our existence was shot through with it. It set in motion trains of circumstances which brought us misfortune we felt we didn't deserve. But did not we, ourselves, set the ball rolling? Sometimes we think fear out to be classed with stealing. It seems to cause more trouble."

- Alcoholics Anonymous

As long as we live in fear and insecurity, we'll reside inside a codependent paradigm where we continually seek something outside of ourselves, such as a relationship to provide us with a sense of security, and validation, to make us feel okay. This fear and insecurity are steeped in a sense of being incomplete. If we don't feel whole and complete within ourselves, we will often look to relationships, career success, romance, shopping, gambling, etc. to prop ourselves up, making us feel whole. This kind of inadequacy, and the anxiety that accompanies it, leaves us vulnerable to addictions, abusive relationships, and a countless variety of illnesses both mental and physical.

Our freedom, independence, and health depend upon the identification and elimination of our false dependencies. Although it's perfectly normal to love our families and participate in them, we must make sure that we do so within healthy boundaries. I cannot emphasize enough the importance of humanizing our family members and our parents, instead of them and sacrificing our own well-being in trying to meet their needs over our own.

"Even as adults, we do not gain freedom of choice until we see the past clearly and experience our feelings about it."
  - Kenneth M. Adams

In the example of Dorothy, her desire to leave the family farm and build a life outside of and away from her family or origin aroused such great anxiety and insecurity within her that she decided not to leave and instead condemned herself to a life of mediocrity on a farm where she clearly did not want to live.

The love and support that we extend to our families must be born of an authentic desire and not of obligation. There is no freedom in obligation. Obligation breeds resentment. We must be willing to examine ourselves, our relationship to our families, our culture, and even our religion of origin to then determine who we choose to be rather than remaining obedient to a role that was assigned to us without our consent. We must find the courage to discover ourselves beyond the boundaries of who we were allowed to be in the presence of our families.

Let's look at individuation and independence, as well as how these are connected to setting and maintaining healthy boundaries.

Webster's dictionary defines individuation as: the process by which individuals in society become differentiated from one another.

When I refer to individuation, I'm talking about how we become differentiated from our parents and our families, cultures, and religions of origin.

One of my favorite quotes by Socrates is, *"the unexamined life is not worth living."* I love this quote because it challenges an individual to move beyond the comfort of the automatic, of the expected, and to look beyond the status quo.

In order for us to be the most authentic version of ourselves, we have to experience being the author of our own life. For example, I cannot say that I'm Catholic just because I was born that way. I have to discover Catholicism newly, for myself, in order to own it and really be part of it. To be empowered in our lives as an adult, we must choose the life that we're living, not just go along with something predestined for us by someone else.

By exploring and examining our family of origin dynamics, our culture and/or religion of origin, and the roles, rules, and expectations, that come with them, we get to then choose to align ourselves with that culture/religion/etc. or not.

Here's one example of cultural expectations and how they subtly impact our choices, potentially sabotaging our deepest desires. I cannot tell you how many women I've worked with whose hearts' secret desire is to be a stay-at-home mom.

They dream of getting married, setting up housekeeping, making babies, baking cookies, crafting, and strolling Junior through the park in the afternoon with the sunlight beaming down on their face.

They dream of baby showers, toddler birthday parties, and moms' coffee clutches. They dream of husbands who work hard, are successful, and provide for them financially.

Those are the dreams that are buried deep within their hearts. However, they were born in the United States of America in a culture that screams feminism with a bias for feminism being interpreted as a woman who values and wouldn't dream of sacrificing her career for family. We raise our young women to become educated so that they can secure great careers with unlimited earning potential. We don't teach them to take a class on child development alongside that statistics course. We don't emphasize the importance of prudent household management, nor do we assign great value to the fine art of domestic engineering. We don't raise women to lean into their femininity and softness, we raise them to compete with men in the workforce. Our culture teaches them to be hypersexualized, aggressive, outspoken, and financially independent.

Don't get me wrong, I believe it's extremely important for women to be educated, financially independent, and sexually aware. I am not recommending that we move back into the dark ages of women being barefoot and pregnant in the kitchen. However, we should not feel embarrassed for wanting something beyond a career. In fact, we shouldn't feel obligated to have one if we don't want one. What happened to choice?

A woman shouldn't be embarrassed to be a domestic engineer. A woman shouldn't be embarrassed to meet her husband in college, get married, become a wife and mother rather than an executive utilizing her degree. There will be plenty of time for her to use that degree once her children are in school full time or grown and out of the house. Why should she be condemned for choosing to spend those precious years when her children are small and need her most, at home? She should not feel embarrassed about this but instead, honored, supported, and empowered to make such a choice.

On the opposite side of the spectrum, there are women who choose to be childless. I happen to be one of those women. I can tell you from first-hand experience how much prejudice, criticism, and judgment I have received over this choice. When people, and when I say people I'm talking about strangers, people I've met in the mall or standing in line at Starbucks, ask me if I have children and I answer no - I cannot tell you how many times the response was a gasp coupled with an admonishment warning me that I am making a mistake and encouraging me to reconsider lest I regret my poor decision in the future, once I've passed through menopause and it's too late. Gratefully, I live in the United States. I am a sovereign woman and I have choices. I have the courage to live my truth and know that I cannot please everyone. I must stand tall in my wholeness and power. I choose to live my life on my terms.

There is no place like home. So where is home? What if instead of home being an address, or a group of people that I may or may not be related to, home was that place of wholeness and sovereignty within myself? What if, what Dorothy was searching for, that she thought was back home in Kansas, was really within herself? Like Glenda the Good Witch said: *"you've always had the power my dear, you just had to learn it for yourself."* What if that power wasn't in returning to a location, the family farm, but in building a home wherever you are?

Let's look at what happens when we do not own our power. When we think that home is somewhere outside of ourselves.

In my many years of being a coach and mentoring people during early sobriety, one of the repeating reasons for failure in a client's recovery program is their hesitation, or unwillingness, to betray their family system.

I've seen this happen more time than I can count. Here's a common example: A person is in treatment for substance abuse or a mental health issue, and their treatment is concluding. Their case manager is busy trying to help them put together a post-treatment plan and the client states that they want to go home.

Even under the best of circumstances, meaning the client has a loving, healthy family that supports their recovery, families are overwhelmed with their own responsibilities and personal/professional obligations. They've not had the time or training to become mental health/substance abuse experts to professionally guide their family member through the next phase of their development. Not to mention, they have no way of anticipating or controlling the environmental triggers that will undoubtedly arise upon the client's return to their original surroundings. The places they used, acted out, and all the people who're still there, living that same lifestyle, that are all too willing to encourage the client to relapse. Nor is it their job to do any of the above.

Healthy young adults' graduate high school, go off to college, get a job, and their own place to live. It should be no different with someone graduating a treatment program. They can move into a sober or transitional living environment. They can find a sober roommate, get a job, and continue with their recovery.

Although it is possible for family members to participate in the recovery process and make changes to the family system, I've found that this is extremely rare. Typically, they've not done any work on themselves and therefore continue to perpetuate a dysfunctional structure of codependency, addiction, and or other sicknesses no different than the ones that guided the client into the person they became with the habits, neuroses, and challenges they possessed. In those instances, it's a disaster to return home.

In these cases, clients are implored not to return home but to instead move into a transitional living situation that has structure, and healthy leadership. An environment that will help them continue with their recovery work, assisting them in obtaining employment, and encouraging them to continue to actively participate with their recovery community.

It's imperative for these individuals to maintain their distance and create new homes. Homes within themselves. Homes that are now based on health, recovery, and interdependence.

In 1986 Melanie Beattie wrote a book entitled *Codependent No More*, that started an important conversation in our culture about codependency and boundaries. In 1991 Kenneth Adams took the subject even further delving into the topic of enmeshment. illuminating a concept known as emotional incest. In his book, *Silently Seduced: When Parents Make Their Children Partners*, Dr. Adams shares the experiences of victims of covert parental abuse and the impacts of growing up in a dysfunctional home.

Covert Abuse vs. Overt Abuse

Overt abuse is much more easily identified because it is quantifiable. If someone is beaten or molested that's clear and obvious. But what if the abuse being experienced isn't physical violence? What if there was subtle alcoholism? Meaning your parent wasn't falling down drunk, but they were under the influence enough that they were obviously not present in your life. Perhaps they were busy sipping scotch in their office while doing paperwork and ignoring you? Again, very subtle but make no mistake, neglect, and emotional abandonment are just as devastating as being physically assaulted and can have long-term negative effects.

Now let's look at the other extreme. What about those who suffered from a parent's love that felt more confining than freeing, more demanding than giving, more intrusive the nurturing. Often those children became trapped in a psychological marriage with that parent. This form of covert enmeshed abuse is not so easily identified.

Jordan Peterson, a celebrated clinical psychologist says, *"Sometimes the reason that you are suffering is that you won't let go of the thing that is biting you."* The sense of obligation and necessity we have, to remain over-involved with our abusers, is problematic. It doesn't matter if the person biting us or impeding our growth and happiness, is our blood relative or parent, they DO NOT have the right to do so. Until we set a boundary and stop allowing it and or sever communication completely, we'll continue being eaten alive.

Consider, a young adult who's working hard waiting tables for minimum wage to put themselves through college but is constantly being asked for money by a parent who's suffering from substance abuse issues

119

or untreated mental health issues and refuses to seek help or a job of their own.

What about the child who earns a full scholarship to attend school out of state but turns down the opportunity because his moms thinks it's too far away, and she needs him here, at home?

Culturally we do a poor job because we encourage this behavior. We praise children who stay home to care for their families, instead of pursuing a life and dreams of their own. There is a BIG difference between a child who was raised lovingly and selflessly, is now an executive in a very empowered financial circumstance, and desires to freely contribute to his parent financially as a loving gesture, not out of obligation, and a parent who's holding a child financially hostage by leveraging their neediness and emotional connection, making demands that the child has no power to resist.

One of my favorite Ken Adams quotes is, *"There's nothing loving or caring about a close parent-child relationship when it services the needs and feelings of a parent rather than the child."*

I cannot tell you how many young men I've encountered who are so controlled by their mothers financially and emotionally that they are suffocating, yet cannot or will not let go, even though it's costing them their virility, vitality, and independence. It's truly heartbreaking.

We've looked at how children can be enmeshed with their parents but what about when a child is holding their parent hostage? This doesn't necessarily need to be a child/parent relationship, it could also be a cousin and a grandparent, or any other combination of family members trying to help.

Let's look at the ways we enable substance abuse and mental illness in our family systems.

Young adults or family members of any age can truly be disastrous. I know of countless family members who thought they were being helpful, allowing a family member who struggled with mental illness and or substance abuse to move in with them, only to be held hostage energetically by someone who was unwell, untreated, and or unwilling to take their medication. Unfortunately, many of these scenarios end in tragedy.

For example, at the time of this books' publication, one of the most recent tragedies shaking our country has been the Uvalde, Texas shooting. The massacre was the act of a troubled young man who had a history of developmental/behavioral issues that had transitioned into serious mental health challenges. His behavior had gotten progressively worse and more aggressive as he got older. His social media accounts and interactions with peers provided clear evidence of his unstable, inappropriate conduct, and penchant for violence.

After reading many of the published statements from his parents and family members, it's clear that they lacked a comprehensive understanding of their son's mental health issues. His Grandmother, lacking a clear picture of who her grandson had become, invited him to live with her, in her home. I cannot imagine that she had any idea that he would steal and crash her car, after shooting her in the face and nearly taking her life.

One of my favorite sayings that I share with many of my own clients is, *"you can have a rattlesnake for a pet, as long as you don't treat it like a bunny rabbit."*

How many times do we allow ourselves to slip into denial about our loved ones because we cannot bear to face the reality of what it means to be honest? How many times do we put bunny ears on rattlesnakes only to wind up getting bit or injured?

Judy Morris

Domestic violence is unlike any other crime. It does not happen in a vacuum. It does not happen because someone is in the wrong place at the wrong time. Our families and homes are meant to be our safe place, our sanctuary. This is one of the reasons that this form of violence is so difficult to face. Because it's violence at the hands of someone we know, from someone we love and who claims to love us. Domestic Violence does not only happen between spouses or lovers. Webster's Dictionary defines domestic violence as, *"violent or abusive behavior directed by one family or household member against another."* Often, it's the person who's supposed to be our nurturer (parent) who's become the perpetrator. In either case, because these horrors are taking place within the home, the incidents are cloaked in shame, and then buried away. In many cases, physical violence is far less damaging than emotional and verbal violence. The loud voices of blaming, shaming, and condemnation shape the innocent minds of children causing lasting damage and difficulty in their future relationships including social, professional, and personal/romantic dysfunction. Domestic violence rips through the fabric of the victim's life. The psychological, emotional, and social impacts of domestic violence can linger long after the violence has subsided, and even after the victim has separated from their perpetrator.

The US Department of Justice estimates that 1.3 million women and 835,000 men are victims of physical violence by an intimate partner each year.

The NCADV also reports that among all domestic violence victims, 85% are women; on average, one in every four American women will experience domestic violence in her lifetime. Crime statistics also indicate that close to one-third of all female homicide victims were killed by an intimate partner.

According to the National Center for PTSD, there are several scenarios that may indicate an unhealthy relationship, when one partner:

- Has complete control of all household finances
- Limits or completely closes off the other partner's social life
- Isolates the other partner from friends and family
- Consistently threatens to ruin the reputation of the other partner
- Repeatedly tries to scare the other by breaking things, punching holes in the wall, and hurting or threatening to hurt pets
- Systematically evokes feelings of guilt or shame in the other partner

We live in a culture that deifies the family unit, sending a subliminal message of loyalty at all costs to family members. Victims are encouraged to stay and try to work things out. Our judicial system has a very lax way of dealing with domestic violence giving perpetrators a mere slap on the wrist, such as a small fine or a few days in jail after a brutal assault. It's obvious and tragic that law enforcement treats domestic violence as an inconvenience, a "domestic dispute," rather than the criminal act that it is.

A common question we often ask is, "Why people would choose to stay in an abusive situation or relationship?"

Stockholm Syndrome, which is often assumed to be only between hostage holders and their victims can also be found in family, romantic, and interpersonal relationships. The abuser may be a husband or wife, boyfriend or girlfriend, father or mother, or any other role in which the abuser is in a position of control or authority.

It's important to understand the components of Stockholm Syndrome as they relate to abusive and controlling relationships. Once the syndrome is understood, it's easier to recognize why victims support, love, and often even defend their abusers and controllers.

Judy Morris

Every syndrome has symptoms or behaviors, and Stockholm Syndrome is no exception. While a clear-cut list has not been established due to varying opinions by researchers and experts, a few of the key behaviors that are most common are included below:

- Positive feelings by the victim toward their abuser/controller
- Negative feelings by the victim toward family, friends, or authorities that may be trying to rescue/support them or win their release
- Support of the abuser's reasons and behaviors
- Positive feelings by the abuser toward the victim
- Supportive behaviors by the victim, at times, helping their abuser
- Inability to engage in behaviors that may assist in their release or detachment

A victim of Stockholm Syndrome irrationally clings to the notion that if only they try hard enough and love the person unconditionally, their abuser will eventually see the light. The abuser, in turn, encourages that false hope for as long as they desire in order to string their victim along. Seeing that the abuser can sometimes behave well, the victim often blames themselves for the times when their partner mistreats them. Because their life has been reduced to a single goal and dimension which subsumes everything else – they will dress, work, cook, and perform sexually in ways that please the narcissistic partner. The victim's self-esteem becomes exclusively dependent upon their abuser's approval and hypersensitive to their disapproval.

When discussing psychopaths and narcissists however, they can never be pleased. Relationships with them are always about control, and never about mutual love. Consequently, the more a psychopath gets from their partners, the more they demand from them. Any person who makes it their life objective to satisfy a psychopathic partner is therefore bound to eventually suffer from a lowered self-esteem. After years of mistreatment, they may feel too discouraged and depressed to leave their abuser. The psychopath may have damaged their self-esteem to the point where they feel that they wouldn't be attractive to anyone else. Dr, Joseph Carver calls this distorted perception of reality a *"cognitive dissonance,"* which psychopaths commonly inculcate in their victims.

"The combination of 'Stockholm Syndrome' and 'cognitive dissonance produces a victim who firmly believes the relationship is not only acceptable but also desperately needed for their survival. The victim feels they would mentally collapse if the relationship ended. In long-term relationships, the victims have invested everything and 'placed all their eggs in one basket.' The relationship now decides their level of self-esteem, self-worth, and emotional health."

- Dr. Joseph Carver

Corporate Stockholm Syndrome is also alive and well in organizations where a boss or supervisor has a similar type of control over an employee. Typically, there's a carrot dangling in front of the employee who believes that they'll eventually benefit if they are compliant. Many are "frozen" into their roles because they lack the energy or self-esteem to move on or seek a change of scenery. Like hamsters on a treadmill, they work for the captor who feeds them scraps of kindness intermittently while keeping them under the influence with their control tactics.

The only way to escape this kind of dangerous dependency is to remove ourselves permanently from the influence of our abuser. Any contact with them keeps us trapped in their web of manipulation and deceit. In some respects, however, this is a circular proposition. If we have the strength to leave and the clarity of mind to reconsider our relationship with them, then we're probably not suffering from Stockholm Syndrome. We may have been temporarily lost in the fog of the trauma bond. But those who do suffer from Stockholm Syndrome often find themselves lost in a dark tunnel. They find themselves so far down the tunnel there is no more light. If and when they wake up to what's going on, they will need to enlist the aid of a professionally trained therapist who is an expert on the topic, to be able to help to tell the truth about what's happened and take the necessary actions to save themselves.

Escaping From Unhealthy Relational Dynamics

First and foremost, we must recognize that no one is coming to save us. We are the one we've been waiting for. We must come to the realization that we are worthy of kindness and safety - no matter what external messages we've been receiving. And once we connect to that ray of hope we must nurture it into a strong sense of positive self-regard.

It's so important to nurture and preserve our positive self-regard to be able to recognize any form of abuse regardless of who may be perpetrating it. When we lose that, we become vulnerable to abuse in all its forms.

What if we have never had a positive self-regard? What if we've grown up in an environment that was dysfunctional and abusive?

One of the most difficult memories of my own childhood was watching my mother become the victim of narcissistic abuse. I witnessed her captor manipulating her slowly over time by promising her all of the things she dreamed of. I saw the insanity, the intensity, and the drama. She had been worn down in so many ways. She was working full-time, in addition to her gigs as a performer on the weekends. She was miserable in a dead-end marriage, with an older man who had little earning potential and no interest in being a parent to me, her teenage daughter. Her soon-to-be love interest saw her weakness, knew her dreams, and took the opportunity to strike. I hated all of it. Every moment of it. But I was 13 years old and was powerless to change anything.

I remember coming home one night after being with friends and feeling like I was walking into World War 3. Things were being broken and thrown, there was screaming and violence. I picked up my brother, who was a toddler at the time, and very calmly walked next door to our neighbor's house to call the police. By the time the police arrived, they'd already resolved their dispute and calmed down. My mother denied my allegations, explaining to the police that I was an emotional teenager who was overacting. The police let it go at that. They didn't bother to ask me any questions. They had no interest in my statement because I was a child and after all, it was only a domestic dispute to be handled among the adults. Adults that lacked the self-regulation and maturity to handle their emotions and disputes in appropriate ways. Instead, they created an emotionally hazardous environment of instability and chaos.

I had SO much judgment toward my mother, but that judgment was replaced with compassion when I found myself in a similar situation. I swore I would never end up in a relationship like that, but I did. Children live what they learn, and by the time I was 18 years old I found myself in a dysfunctional relationship with a man who violated me in ways that I had never before or since experienced. There was verbal abuse in the form of insults, threats, and intimidation, but believe it or not, the most traumatizing part was the stalking.

I actually encouraged him to be a private investigator because he could so skillfully break into anyplace, find anything, and anyone, and this was before cell phones and instant access to things via the internet. It was terrifying. I haven't seen that man in over 20 years, but I still look over my shoulder and check the locks multiple times when I'm home alone. I've never been able to live on the ground floor of a building, or leave my windows open after an incident where he broke into my apartment and tried to kill my boyfriend, long after we had broken up. He hurt me in ways I didn't know I could be hurt, playing upon my vulnerabilities and insecurities in predatory ways. I am eternally grateful to have escaped and that he finally left me in peace. Many other women were not as lucky.

I am so grateful that I chose to get help. I chose to get sober. I chose to go to therapy. I chose to stop hurting myself and to start living.

I want you to know something - EVERY SINGLE HUMAN BEING ON THIS PLANET has an inalienable right to exist in an environment that is free from abuse and harassment. All it takes is a moment to make the decision that you want to exercise that right and choose to take the necessary actions to pursue it.

We must understand that we cannot put people on pedestals. We cannot make acceptations or excuses for family members, lovers, friends, or employers who are treating us abusively. We must find the courage to tell the truth to ourselves and like the famous airline example, we must put the mask on ourselves first before we help our neighbor.

If you are living in an abusive or dysfunctional situation and cannot afford therapy, you can begin the healing process by educating yourself. We live in a time where we have access to information like never before. If we remain ignorant it's because we've chosen to remain that way. We don't have to spend a small fortune to learn. We can take the small step of educating ourselves.

There are libraries filled with books, we can go there and read, we have smartphones and computers. There are so many incredibly generous mental health professionals who publish educational content for free on their social media platforms and blogs. And there are all kinds of peer support groups, and community organizations available to help.

There are endless videos available on YouTube and other media platforms. Two of the best tools I've found and continue to use today, are prayer and meditation, both are powerful, and both are free. Studies have shown that daily mindful meditation practices produce measurable changes in the regions of our brains that are associated with memory, sense of self, empathy, and stress.

No matter where you come from, it is possible to live an empowered, enlivened, and vibrant life of emotional and physical health.

It's said that pain is the touchstone of spiritual growth. And no one knows that pearl of wisdom better than those of us who come from painful beginnings.

Speaking of pearls - a natural pearl forms when an irritant works its way into a particular species of oyster, mussel, or clam. As a defense mechanism, the mollusk secretes a fluid to coat the irritant. Layer upon layer of this coating is deposited on the irritant until a lustrous pearl is formed. As with pearls so it can be with people. We can transform the irritants/pain from our childhoods into lustrous pearls of growth, wisdom, maturity, and spirituality IF we chose to.

I know that it's only by working through the challenges that I faced in my own upbringing and early adulthood that I've been able to become the woman I am today. I would not have had the passion, interest, or insight to be the intuitive, committed coach that I have become had I not had a mess to turn into a message.

Only by embracing my pain and accepting the reality of what happened in my life was I able to grieve my childhood, heal my pain, discover/develop my unique gifts/talents to the world, and trust in my purpose to help liberate others.

As I have stated in previous chapters, although I am powerless over what happened in my past, I am not powerless over who I am going to be in the face of it. Acceptance is freedom. Once I accepted life on life's terms and processed my pain, I was able to let go of self-defeating/negative thoughts. I was able to stop comparing myself to others and despairing over what they had or have. By letting go of that which no longer served me, I was able to create a whole new world to live in.

As I have developed my own deep spiritual practice, I've discovered that the Universe is loving and benevolent. Nothing is happening to me, but for me. I no longer have to manipulate circumstances to fit my perfectionistic views and prove my worth. I now operate from a place of wholeness and worthiness. I have faith that the Universe is conspiring in my favor and trust that everything is working out perfectly. I'm willing and able to listen and learn these lessons instead of being angry about being a student of life.

Judy Morris

Trust The Process

We are not objects to be owned and managed. We were born to experience all that life has to offer.

A soul is not unlike a seed. It contains within it all the potential to become itself. There are things we can choose like what color we want to paint our house or what car we want to drive, but we do not get to choose whether we are an oak tree or a rose. That's already imprinted in the seed and will unfold organically after being planted in fertile soil.

This is why it's so harmful to try and tell people who they can love. I knew that I liked boys from a very early age. If I had been told that I had to like girls instead, I would have experienced confusion, frustration, and feelings of unease. It would have gone against my nature. I've been studying people and giving advice since I was old enough to talk. The distinction of being a coach was already inside me before I had even discovered it. Therefore, it's equally harmful to try and tell someone what they should do professionally, since there is already a fire somewhere inside of them that's just waiting to be stoked and have its flames fanned by the love and support of their family. There is a great saying attributed to Leo Buscaglia, *"Your talent is the Universe's gift to you. What you do with it is your gift back to the Universe."*

People whose parents come from impoverished backgrounds and have not been to college, often idealize higher education and do everything in their power to push their children toward an advanced degree. Perpetuating a false idea that a degree is a guarantee of employment, financial security, and therefore success is an antiquated superstition that will create false hope, disappointment, and ultimately resentment against the workplace and perhaps even the family that enforced it. Not to mention the hefty loans that will remain as a constant reminder for years to come. What was true seven decades ago, is no longer the truth today. We reside in an age of advanced technology, post-COVID remote work, and empowered entrepreneurialism. We need to focus on a new set of skills that cannot be found in a trade school or even in a basic college education. We are desperately lacking in soft skills such as communication, conflict resolution, teamwork, collaboration, and project management. We're equally lacking in empowered leadership, accountability, and the ability to empower others. I've spent the last decade working with clients on their careers and I can tell you that a degree is no guarantee of anything. I've worked closely with people who possess advanced degrees yet absolutely disdain the industry they've been trained in and can no longer face working within it. I've seen people over-educated with countless certificates and degrees, yet no soft skills to speak of. People who cannot find their voice and cannot communicate successfully in an interview.

We've all heard the term starving artist. No parent wants their child to starve, so they will often diminish their child's talent for painting or music as an interesting and entertaining personal characteristic that will never pay a mortgage or secure a retirement plan, demeaning the child's natural inclinations toward anything that doesn't fit the parents' limited view of what will provide security.

Take for example, JK Rowling, the skilled author of the Harry Potter book series. Growing up, her parents did NOT want her to write, to the extent that they deemed her, *"overactive imagination as an amusing personal quirk that would never pay a mortgage or secure a pension."*

Parents who confuse their fear with love, and their desire to protect, block their child's natural, intuitive process from organically developing into the bright light that their creator intended them to be.

The truth of the matter is that we cannot protect another person from life and there is no such thing as security. Life in and of itself is filled with risk. Risks that we cannot control. So, the only thing we can do is manage those risk. And we can teach our children to do the same. We cannot save them from the trials and tribulations of life.

"Don't worry about the future or worry but know that worrying is as effective as trying to solve an algebra equation by chewing Bubble gum - the real troubles in your life are apt to be things that never crossed your worried mind the kind that blindsides you at 4 p.m. on some idle Tuesday."

- Baz Luhrmann

Khalil Gibran, a Lebanese American Poet famously wrote:

"...Your children are not your children
They are the sons and daughters of life's longing for itself
They come through you but not from you
And though they are with you, yet they belong not to you
You may give them your love but not your thoughts
For they have their own thoughts
You may house their bodies but not their souls
For their souls dwell in the house of tomorrow
Which you cannot visit, not even in your dreams
You may strive to be like them
But seek not to make them like you
For life goes not backward, nor tarries with yesterday..."

We want to secure the future, of ourselves, our children, our families, and our interests. So, we seek to control, in pursuit of success and happiness. We give so much power to our circumstances, falling prey to the false belief that we can wrest satisfaction and happiness out of this world if only we manage it well. However, life is not to be controlled, it is to be lived. And one of the most valuable lessons we can teach our children is how to live life well. How to live life on life's terms because we cannot prepare the road for them. It is our job to prepare them for the road.

We are inhabitants of a benevolent Universe and life was not meant to be fraught with so much struggle. There is an ease that comes when we flow with the stream of life. Unfortunately, rather than focusing on learning the laws of the Universe and how to live in harmony with them, we live in a society that prizes material success and achievement above connection and experience. There is a Frankensteinian obsession to usurp the laws of the Universe and rise above God himself. We are failing at that pursuit and that failure is coming at a great cost. The destruction of the planet by exploitation of natural resources, pollution, and global warming. Self-importance, grandiosity, and the demise of human connection, increased violence coupled with warped family relations, and an obsession with status and fame.

We are chasing a standard that we are supposed to live up to - what is and is not acceptable. Cultures and religions condemn those who are in same-sex relationships causing even further separation. I am not diminishing the power or necessity of a moral compass — however, that compass no longer serves its purpose when it becomes a mechanism of power to control others.

Inauthenticity, shame, and embarrassment are unique to the human experience. Those emotions are comparison based in an attempt to make others more like ourselves and reduce the anxiety of perceived isolation and separateness.

This is something unique to humans. You do not see this in nature. No oak tree is crying because it is shorter than another oak tree. No rose is harming itself because it isn't as red or pretty as another rose. A squirrel is not invalidated that he is not a tiger. The squirrel is too busy living his best life, going from tree to tree collecting acorns. One of my favorite sayings by Albert Einstein is, *"Everybody is a genius. But if you judge a fish by its ability to climb a tree, it will live its whole life believing that it is stupid."*

You exist; therefore, I exist——that's how the ego is born. French psychoanalyst Jacques Lacan developed the concept of the 'Mirror Stage' to describe the phenomenon when a child begins to distinguish the 'self' and others——encountering one's image in the mirror makes us realize we are autonomous.

The ego is born out of fear and isolation. It creates our identity and separates us from those around us when we were a child. Our ego not only blinds us but also makes others blind. We want to impose our perspective upon others——whatever we see; we want others to see too because we believe our vision of the world is the world. Because we desire so strongly to be right, we attempt to prove our expertise by gaining the agreement of others.

The only way to have our ego function in a healthy way is to develop self-awareness. When we have our ego vs. it having us.

Tasha Eurich, an organizational psychologist, completed research which shows that self-awareness is the foundation for high performance, smart choices, and lasting relationships. It also shows that most people don't see themselves as clearly as they could. "Our data reveals that 95 percent of people believe they are self-aware, but the real number is 12 to 15 percent," she says. "That means, on a good day, about 80 percent of people are lying about themselves——to themselves."

As we pursue winning the game of life by becoming the one who is the most attractive, has the most money, is smarter/better educated, morally superior, and stronger, we are shadowed by a persistent sense of weariness and self-doubt. The ego likes security, certainty, and repetition. It makes us feel comfortable by reinforcing an idealized version of ourselves. If people threaten that illusion, we turn them into an enemy. That's why ego-driven people engage in constant battles—they want to protect the fragile fantasy of who they are. The ego's relentless pursuit of attention and power undermines the goal we want to achieve. Dealing with an unhealthy ego is exhausting.

Let's look at how cognitive dissonance exacerbates an unhealthy ego. Cognitive dissonance describes the mental discomfort that results from holding two conflicting beliefs, values, or attitudes. We tend to seek consistency in our attitudes and perceptions, so this conflict causes feelings of unease or discomfort.

Cognitive dissonance can make us feel anxious and uncomfortable, particularly if the disparity between our beliefs and behaviors involves something that is central to our sense of self. For example, behaving in ways that are not aligned with our personal values may result in intense feelings of discomfort. Our behavior contradicts not just the beliefs we have about the world, but also the beliefs that we have about ourselves.

As William Shakespeare so eloquently stated: *"The lady doth protest too much."* The line, from Hamlet, is spoken by Queen Gertrude in response to the insincere overacting of another character in an attempt to prove his uncle's guilt in the murder of his father.

We need to consider the part within ourselves that feels a need to eradicate or kill off something, often born from the need to disconnect from something that we are afraid or ashamed to be connected to.

Perhaps we see so much violence against the LGBTQ community because those individuals who have buried or hidden a queer part of themselves feel the need to kill it off externally by harming the very thing that reveals them to themselves. Or even worse, a parent who is so driven by external validation that they would disown their own child to look better in the face of their cultural or religious community.

Just like the acorn is destined to become a tree, so are we destined to become our true selves. As discussed in other chapters, when we deify our families, cultures, or religions we are at risk of abandoning our true selves which brings about significant sometimes tragic costs.

Maladaptive coping mechanisms that many people employ to cope with their discomfort include:

- Adopting beliefs or ideas to help justify or explain away the conflict between our beliefs or behaviors. This can sometimes involve blaming other people or outside factors and is often the case when spouses have affairs. An affair is often an attempt to save a marriage by getting ones needs met outside of it, because without those needs being met, they would feel the desire to leave the marriage fully.

- Hiding our beliefs or behaviors from other people. We may feel ashamed of our conflicting beliefs and behaviors, thus hiding that disparity from others can help to minimize feelings of shame and guilt. An example of this is someone hiding their sexuality otherwise known as being in the closet.

- Only seeking out information that confirms our existing beliefs. This phenomenon, known as the confirmation bias, affects the ability to think critically about a situation but helps minimize feelings of dissonance. An example of this is a racist only reading racist materials or following other racist leaders.

Perhaps cultural and religious beliefs are so powerful because we were indoctrinated into them by our caregivers at a young and impressionable age. Our little hearts and minds were so fertile that they readily absorbed the beliefs of our caregivers. How terrifying must it be when we grow up only to discover that our authentic self's conflict with those beliefs? This is part of the problem I see with people who profess to be Christians. Christianity is based on the teachings of Jesus Christ, and Christ's message can be boiled down to one word. Love.

During the last supper, Jesus gave his disciples a new commandment and that commandment, *"A new commandment I give unto you, that you love one another, as I have loved you. By this shall men know you are my disciples if you have love one to another."*

So, what happened to love? Love has devolved into a feeling. It's become confused with the experience of agreement and pleasure. It's as warped and immature a perception as that of a child who imagines the key to happiness being a world in which they could spend their days wandering amusement parks, eating cotton candy and chocolate cake - never having to go to school or perform chores.

Love is a verb, not a noun. Love is an action. Webster's Dictionary defines love as, "unselfish loyal and benevolent concern for the good of another." We have become so concerned with being loved by others that we have forgotten how to be loving toward others. We have become so consumed with getting what we want, that we've forgotten how to give.

There are so many paradoxes in this life. Early in my recovery, I learned that spiritual principles are quite often paradoxical in nature and have included a few of my favorites below.

- **Surrender.** — The word surrender doesn't exactly conjure images of winning. In a 12-step program, only after we've hit rock bottom in despair can we find the humility to surrender and achieve sobriety which we've never been able to accomplish. For me, it was a transformational experience to discover that the moment I admitted powerlessness over alcohol was the very moment I gained power over alcohol and NEVER had to drink it again.

- **We have to give it away to keep it.** - Another statement that doesn't elicit feelings of success. How can it be possible to keep something that you've given away? When we recognize what we've been so freely given, we realize that we cannot afford to not give it away. The only way to know that we have power is in our ability to empower others. If we cannot empower others, we need to look at where we are still operating from a place of fear and disempowerment.

- **Pain is the touchstone of spiritual growth**. – In the example of a caterpillar becoming a butterfly, one must know that disturbing a caterpillar inside its cocoon or chrysalis risks botching their entire transformation. No one can go through this process on its behalf. It's an inside job. The struggle that a caterpillar encounters allows them to build the muscles necessary to sprout wings and become a beautiful butterfly. We too cannot escape the pain of our own transformation. It is for us too, an inside job. We cannot escape the regret, and remorse that inevitably touches each of our lives – not to mention the shame and embarrassment we feel when we review our unbecoming conduct in days gone by. We are spiritual beings having a human experience. We must strive for progress, not perfection.

- **It is by dying that one awakens to eternal life.** – As described above, the caterpillar must die to become a butterfly. In the famous prayer constructed by St. Francis we discover *"it is* *better to give than to receive and that one must die in order to awaken to eternal life.* "Those of us who've worked the steps in a recovery program know that the ego must die, in fact, many of us must experience multiple ego deaths before we're able to build a new character with no reference to the old. The old self must die for a new self to be reborn. This transformation process happens repeatedly in a person's life as we progress on our spiritual journey to self-actualization.

What if we related to ourselves as an infinite expression of the divine, brought to the earth at this specific moment in time to contribute our unique gifts to the world? What if we were not put here to be served, but to serve?

How would that impact our experience of being with others? We cannot learn to love and accept others until we have learned to love and accept ourselves. As stated above, we must give it away to keep it. But we cannot transmit something we haven't got. We cannot abandon ourselves by trying to become what we think society expects us to be. This only leaves us unfulfilled and attempting to compensate by engaging in self-centered behaviors.

We think we came here without a manual or a guide, but this isn't true. Our Higher Power equipped us with something called the emotional guidance system, a GPS for our soul. Why do you think that little voice comes to you when you're doing something contrary to your true self? This little voice, which my dear friend lovingly refers to as her inner Jiminy Cricket, is the inner compass that lets us know when we are off course. We would benefit in unimaginable ways should we learn how to hear it and work from it.

Imagine that you're in your home, suddenly you smell smoke, and the fire alarm goes off. Now picture yourself going to the fire alarm, disconnecting it, ignoring the smoke, and going back to bed. That sounds ridiculous, doesn't it? But isn't that how most people live their lives? The feeling in our gut that says quit that job, the voice that says, don't get on that plane, or the nudge that says go to the doctor and get that checked out. When we ignore these messages from our higher selves, we are in essence disconnecting the alarm and allowing our lives to burn down around us. If you think I'm exaggerating, look at the countless people around you whose health is in ruins because they're ignoring the little voice begging them to get help, the person who surrenders to amputation rather than giving up sweets and reversing their diabetes, the smoker that ignores the doctor's warnings about COPD and emphysema and continues lighting up, or the alcoholic who justifies their drinking because they go to work every day and are "functioning" but ends up dying of liver failure.

There is really no need to suppress our feelings. Why are we so afraid to feel? Perhaps because we have so many unprocessed feelings (not to mention unprocessed trauma). Perhaps we're afraid that if we allow ourselves to feel, we'll never return from the overwhelming experience.

But we cannot ignore our bodies. The only way out is through. We are stronger than we can possibly imagine. We are not just intellectual beings; we are somatic beings as well. Somatic means relating to or affecting the body. When we live in our minds and disconnect from our physicality, we are forsaking one of our most precious resources, our very own bodies.

In Bessel Van Der Kolk's book entitled, *The Body Keeps the Score*, he shows readers how trauma impacts not only our minds but our bodies. By using modern neuroscience, he demonstrates that trauma physically affects the brain and the body, causing anxiety, rage, and the inability to concentrate. Van Der Kolk goes on to describe how using a combination of traditional therapy and somatic techniques, we can heal and regain control of our bodies, rewiring our brains, and rebuilding our lives.

I know firsthand the damage caused by disconnecting that fire alarm. I did it for years, thinking that by drowning my feelings in a sea of Johnny Walker I could escape the pain. But I discovered that didn't work. Next, I got on my healing journey and focused on talk therapy and step work. Thinking I could intellectualize my way out of my feelings. That didn't work either. Ultimately, I found myself 13 years sober and suicidally depressed. Given my history of depression, I was frustrated and angry. Why wasn't I "well" yet? Why wasn't I "happy?"

Again, to quote our Dr. Van Der Kolk, *my body had kept the score and I was avoiding it at all costs.* I had to choose relapse, kill myself, go on psych meds, or engage in somatic therapy. The process of going into my body and releasing my own stored trauma sent me into a healing crisis and I battled respiratory illness for over 2 years. As someone who had suffered from seasonal asthmatic bronchitis, what I was experiencing through somatic therapy was at an entirely new level. I had smoked cigarettes for 25 years and it was no mistake that when I quit smoking in 2014 and started somatic therapy in 2015 my poor body had loads of trauma and toxicity to release.

Now, before you freak out and think that you can never do your body work because you cannot afford to have a healing crisis, allow me to assure you that each person is able to move at their own pace. Not everyone has to jump in headfirst the way I did. Healing is a VERY personalized choice that must be made prayerfully, and with the consultation of your own treatment team. What I'm sharing is my own story my and experience. I've supported many of my clients through this process with much less violent reactions.

Our Higher Power will NEVER give us more than we can handle, and we can use our emotional guidance system as described above to decide what's best for us. I'd also like to note that I have no judgements against psych meds. I took anti-depressants the very first time I got sober as I mentioned in a previous chapter. I just knew intuitively that at this juncture in my healing journey, psych meds weren't going to be the solution for me. Psychiatric medication can be a godsend and a lifesaver for many people throughout different portions of their healing journey. Again, this is a very personal choice. Never let any person who is not a member of your treatment team advise you on medication.

With the support of a skilled therapist, loving sponsor, spiritual mentor, somatic practitioners, and healers of various kinds it's amazing how comfortable we can become allowing ourselves to bear witness to our feelings. It's thrilling, how interested and aware we can become in hearing the message they're trying to convey. Our emotions are often messengers which signal something important that we need to pay attention to.

Part of processing emotions and feeling includes honoring ourselves, and our body, by giving it what it really needs such as rest, connection, pleasure, and leisure. Sometimes when I'm upset or stressed, one of the things on that list can do wonders in helping me reset. By taking a break and listening to my body, sometimes my body will tell me that it's time to make a change.

When we try to suppress, manage, or control our feelings instead of feeling them, it often leads to more suffering. This can also lead us to use avoidant behaviors to numb ourselves, which is not a sustainable approach. Such behaviors might provide temporary relief but ultimately, they will not solve the underlying problem. Further, using avoidant behavior or maladaptive coping strategies to numb emotions causes us to feel even worse in the long term and can often lead to addictions, or relapse.

Those of us who have used drugs, alcohol, sex, and workaholism, (to name a just a few) to manage and control our emotions can tell you how exhausting it is to constantly try to outrun your emotions. When we're focused on numbing our feelings rather than processing them, we prevent ourselves from living a full and meaningful life. Pain, sadness, frustration, and anger are all normal, natural, and healthy parts of the human experience. Our attempts to suppress these emotions suffocate us and prevent us from leading fulfilling lives. Part of being alive is experiencing the full spectrum of human emotion.

Experiencing our emotions and being vulnerable with those closest to us is a sign of strength, not weakness. Ultimately, the way to heal and move through painful experiences is to let ourselves feel. There are many ways to do this. You can join a peer support group and or participate in therapy. You can create art or a journal. There are so many healthy ways to feel we just must be willing to learn them.

All the ascended masters taught about love. From Christ to Buddha, to Mohammad to Veda Vyasa they all taught about love. Ultimately, that is all any of us want, to love and be loved, yet we're confused as to what's in the way of this experience. The biggest barrier is our own ignorance. We've spent thousands of dollars on academic education yet are spiritually ignorant and emotionally impoverished. We've become so defended and defensive that we can no longer scale the walls around our hearts.

Our fear and stinginess have shrunk our hearts and miniaturized our characters. Western society has so normalized miserly behaviors that we find ourselves dealing with Ebenezer Scrooges who have employees earning less than a living wage and condemning the Tiny Tims of this world to death,

We've become disconnected from ourselves and therefore from each other. We minimize the importance of our own contribution, of our own kindness.

Recently, I went to a local department store in search of cosmetics and met one of the most spectacular human beings on the planet. I'll call him Michael. I've rarely had such a beautiful customer service interaction. The next time I needed my cosmetics, I went back to the same counter in that store, in search of Michael. I let him know how special and wonderful he is, and I could see that it was difficult for him to accept and receive my words. Michael was so moved that as I was leaving, he asked if it might be alright for him to give me a hug.

It saddened me, that someone so special was so unaware of themselves. However, it made me happy that I could tell him, and that maybe just maybe from that encounter he could begin to see that magic in himself.

You matter. You really, really matter. Your contribution matters. People need what you are here to give. If we only knew how vital our contribution would be, we would stop playing around in dead-end jobs, and start pursuing our passion and purpose. The most important thing we can do in life is to be a light in the lives of those we love.

We were not put on this earth to fulfill a self-protective misguided ego agenda. We were put here to learn, grow, and contribute to one another. Once we let go of the obsession to get what we want, became interested in understanding why we're here, and how we can contribute to life, the happier we'll become.

There has never been a time in human history where peoples' wants were more accessible to them, especially in the United States. We have a wealth of advisors, coaches, and schools to educate us in the fine art of desire acquisition. During this time of opulence, prosperity, and access we have never seen more divorce, disease, addiction, mental illness, or depression. Suicide is the third leading cause of death in young people and is the 9th leading cause for adults. If material success was the source of happiness, there would be no overdosed entertainers or millionaires. How many famous people have we seen in the media past and present who had it all and lost it due to suicide or drug addiction?

There is no magic fix that can improve our lives or save us from our unhappiness and there is certainly nothing outside of ourselves that will deliver happiness. Our happiness or lack thereof is directly connected to our self-awareness and state of consciousness. If we are asleep at the wheel of life, we cannot make the necessary changes to help us align with our highest self.

Although no one is coming to save us, we can be our own savior. You are the one you've been waiting for. You can wake up and take action beginning today.

One of my dear friends, who's a brilliant specialist in her field, was withering away in a dead-end corporate job. Through a series of unfortunate events culminating with the sudden death of another friend, she realized that she could no longer live out of alignment with her soul. She had known what her creative destiny was when she was 7 years old, and within the space of a week, she took the leap to manifest it. Now she's a bad-ass creative entrepreneur with two successful businesses, a love filled marriage with her soulmate, and a life she only ever imagined. This choice didn't take a million years or a million dollars. Within a week of her friend passing away, she'd given notice and started her business – if fact, the Universe was so excited that she finally heeded her souls calling that it sent her three big clients before her website was online. If that isn't confirmation, I don't know what is.

We can learn how to love and care for ourselves by living our truth, nurturing our bodies, minds, and spirits, and contributing to others.

If you've read this far then you're ready to live a miraculous life. A life of health, healing, peace, and happiness.

So how does one create a life of miracles? If you pause for a moment and think back on your life, you should be able to recall a time when something happened that was extraordinary - when some divine, cosmic energy seemed to appear out of nowhere to help you in some extraordinary, unexpected, and vital way.

Perhaps you're aware of how you co-created that miracle - by asking for divine intervention or perhaps it seemed to happen without any action on your part. Either way, you can be sure that miracles don't just happen out of the blue. They happen when we become interested in them, when we become present to the possibility of them, and when we become available to them.

It is possible to live a miraculous life. That nagging Groundhog Day feeling inside of you that is dissatisfied with the hamster wheel you are on, going through the motions of a life that you settled for vs. the life of unlimited creativity, self-expression, and fulfillment that you always dreamed of is your soul urging you to take action, to wake up out of the trance of automaticity.

Our creator did not intend miracles to be occasional occurrences in our lives, such as when we have a child, create a grand piece of art, or when we're in immediate need of aid. We were designed to live a miraculous life, where the extraordinary is part of our daily experience.

Let's look at the mechanics of a miracle and how to align ourselves with that divine energy to support us in connecting to our deepest desires.

Judy Morris

What Is a Miracle?

A miracle is "An extraordinary event manifesting divine intervention in human affairs."

From a metaphysical point of view, a miracle is an event that results from the intervention of a higher, unknown law. Nothing just happens. All true action is governed by laws and can be explained by cause and effect. That's the beautiful thing about our Universe — it's governed by laws. When we understand how Universal law works, we can learn how to benefit from them so that we can live in alignment with our deepest desires. When we're in harmony with the Universe, our creative desires are much easier to connect to and manifest. When we're connected to the divine, we're also connected to our higher selves, and when we're connected to our higher selves, we can exist on a higher plane of consciousness - the place of intuitive guidance, peace, and prosperity, living a life of integrity, creativity, connection, and harmony.

As described above, a miracle is an extraordinary event manifesting divine intervention in human affairs. So how do miracles work? In order to manifest a miracle, we must:

- Believe that it is possible
- Have a deep and heart-centered (not ego-centered) desire for it
- Be open and available to it (or to something even better!)
- Take action with integrity toward the miracle we're about to manifest

Using the above mechanics, let's explore a real-life example of how this works.

Judy Morris

As you know, I had a very serious drinking problem. It got to a point where I not only realized I needed to stop, but I really wanted to stop - where in my previous attempts I had not. This time I truly wanted to be sober. I was convinced it was possible because I knew several people who were successfully sober. I had a deep heart-centered desire for it. I didn't want sobriety because it was going to make me look good, get me out of trouble, or help me get what I wanted in life, etc. If I'd wanted to pursue sobriety because of ulterior motives, it would have simply been an ego-driven manipulation and would not have been sustainable. Now, I wanted to be sober for no other reason than the natural consequences that come with it: freedom, improved physical and mental health, and vitality. That's it. It was a heart-centered desire. I was open and available to being blessed with any other gifts that might come in addition to my sobriety, but my desire to be sober wasn't contingent upon such gifts. It was like the old saying goes, "*Virtue is its own reward.*"

Importantly, I was willing to take action with integrity toward the miracle I was seeking. I stopped drinking, regularly attended 12-step meetings, and started receiving guidance from a sober mentor known as a sponsor. I also began to deal with my depression by going to therapy. I was willing to be uncomfortable, to take contrary action, to live in the unknown, and to collaborate with my Higher Power in order to make it happen.

So often I talk with people who want the results but do not want to take action. It's as if they imagine their Higher Power to be like Santa Claus. The logic goes like this: If I am good over a period of time then Santa will bring me presents like my dream career or a perfect relationship. It's incredible to me that some people believe their soulmate will just suddenly appear on their doorstep without any action on their part. Or conversely, some people are hyper-focused on their actions and then get depressed when they don't produce the exact desired outcome.

Unfortunately, these are totally unrealistic expectations. We must instead be in the action business, taking action with integrity toward the miracle we wish to manifest while leaving the results to our Higher Power and the Universe. When we want to manifest a specific miracle, we must energetically align ourselves with that desire and be open and available to it, and then, with confidence, allow the Universe to provide us with that outcome or with something even better.

For most people, this is a tall order. We are such a control-obsessed society that to even think of taking action with integrity and then patiently waiting for the outcome seems inconceivable. When we don't get the job or the relationship that we wanted, it's hard to believe that it's because there is something better for us out there. Or maybe we are not manifesting our miracles because we have more work to do to align ourselves more energetically with our desires.

But that is exactly how it works! We must be willing to take whatever action necessary to align ourselves with the outcome we wish to manifest and then believe with our whole hearts that our Higher Power and the Universe will deliver the exact result for the highest good of all concerned. Remember, all true action is governed by law. Nothing just happens. All happenings can be explained by the law of cause and effect. When we do the right thing for the right reason (if it's for the wrong reason we will not get the same result), we will get the best outcome for the highest good of all concerned. That is metaphysical law. We must let go of our need to know what that is. We need to become invested in our own thoughts, motives, and actions and must believe with our deepest inner knowing that our Higher Power and the Universe will take care of the rest.

Once you start practicing this method in your life and begin to see the miraculous results you won't want to go back to living any other way! I have personally been using this method for over 20 years. I have manifested my recovery from alcoholism and debilitating depression. I have used it in my career to manifest every job I ever wanted. I have also used this method with my clients to manifest the most extraordinary results in their lives, careers, and recovery, and it works without fail.

Our Higher Power and the Universe NEVER fail us. When we use this method, we may not get exactly what we want but always get what we need while we continue to learn and grow. Soon we're able to start operating from a higher state of consciousness, from a place of spirit and true purpose instead of the limiting desires of the ego conjured from our lower nature. And when you begin to operate with spirit and true purpose instead of mere survival it is truly a game-changer.

Heart or Ego?

Modern society has taught us to identify with our ego - I, me, myself - and now self-esteem has become confused with grandiosity. We so strongly identify with self-importance and are so laser-focused on our own intellect that we have become disconnected from our hearts.

One of my favorite definitions of "heart" is "Emotional or moral nature as distinguished from intellectual nature; a generous disposition that reflects compassion, love, affection, courage or enthusiasm, especially when maintained during a difficult situation."

We go to school and spend years learning how to develop our intellect. We are taught to stand out, make things happen, become winners. If our feelings get hurt, we are told to not be so sensitive and to toughen up. There are so many messages in western culture that tell us to hustle, keep our heads down, and not allow our feelings to interfere with hard work. There are not many messages that encourage us to even connect with our hearts let alone follow them, and this imbalance between heart and mind has diverted us from our spiritual development. Without encouragement and guidance on the development of our heart-mind connection, we are deprived of other precious internal assets such as intuition, inspiration, and faith in the organic unfolding of events. There is tremendous value in connecting to our hearts because it is there that our deepest desires reside. When we act from our heart - not our ego — we allow the magic to happen.

But how do we know whether our desire is coming from our heart or our ego?

When something is a heart-centered desire it presents itself softly. It comes as a whisper of intuition. We walk toward it slowly, thoughtfully,

155

respectfully, without wanting to harm anyone in the process. Patience is an innate characteristic that accompanies it.

When something is driven by ego it presents as loud, demanding, impatient, and it is willing to go to any lengths to get the outcome it wants, no matter the cost. Its desire is not for the highest good of all concerned. The ego only desires what is best for itself, no matter what happens to others.

Now that we have a basic understanding of the mechanics of a miracle and have the willingness to manifest one, we must maintain an open mind. This means that we're willing to learn from the process and accept what has not been working in the area of our life in which we're seeking a miracle. Although miracles can and do happen in an instant, sometimes they don't. We must be willing to do this work consistently over a period of time. If we're serious about learning this method of manifestation - as well as a new way to view the world - we must be patient with ourselves and the process.

We must also develop an awareness of the way we've been spending our most valuable asset - the one and only non-renewable resource we have - our time. If we are not putting aside focused time toward self-discovery, we'll need to start examining our priorities. For example, if you have always wanted to start a side hustle and your excuse has been that you don't have time, you will have to begin confronting all the ways you are spending your time such as Netflix bingeing or hanging out with friends.

We all have busy lives and it's easy to blame circumstances for the results (or lack thereof) in our lives. However, living a miraculous life requires that we develop an empowered relationship with ourselves and the world around us. We are the only one responsible for our lives - no one else. No matter what may have happened in the past, we are the ones who must take action to move forward toward our health, healing, and growth. No one can do that for us. No one is coming to rescue us.

You are the one you have been waiting for and you must be willing to embark on the journey of self-discovery to uncover the hidden blocks of self-sabotage, limiting beliefs, unresolved anger, grief, or pain. You must be willing to let go of that which no longer serves you and is impeding the manifestation of miracles in your life. You must also be willing to forgive the past (yourself and others), to break the chains that bind you. As long as you are living in the past (resentment, anger, guilt), you will never be free to walk toward tomorrow which is where all possibility lives.

Accepting life on life's terms isn't always easy. It requires maturity, a willingness to be responsible for one's own life and actions, and a commitment to be deeply grounded in reality. However, the freedom and power that come from that way of living are undeniable and irresistible.

Judy Morris

Dealing with Fear & Insecurity

Have you ever noticed that whenever you commit to a goal, circumstances suddenly arise that seem to sabotage your success? Whenever we create a new possibility, everything in our way eventually gets revealed, clearing the path so that our deepest desires can manifest themselves.

When I first started meditating, I didn't like it. I didn't have a clear understanding of how it worked or how it would help me. Believe me, I read lots of articles on the science and spirituality of it. I understood it conceptually, but I really didn't understand how it applied to me. Every time I would sit down to meditate, I would experience a lot of resistance and discomfort. Therefore, it was no surprise that it took me some time before I was able to accept this practice as a habit.

The problem with my meditation was that rather than leaning into my resistance and looking at it with a desire to learn the lesson it was trying to teach me; I was resisting the uncomfortability of it all and avoiding it. Thankfully, I had an amazing coach who helped me see this and pressed me to journal about what was disturbing me. This helped me to realize that meditation made me uncomfortable because it highlighted the gaps between where I was and where I wanted to be. That's a valuable insight to gain. If we can't see the gaps, if we can't see what's in the way, then we can't make changes. And if nothing changes, nothing changes. Once I saw where the resistance was coming from, I was able to let go and commit to the practice.

In a relatively short period of time, it was revealed to me why this was such a magical and inexplicable practice. I began to notice that I had more peace and presence during my day and that my intuition felt stronger. I also noticed that I had more patience. Instead of saying something angry or responding in an impatient or unkind way to a message, I noticed a pause before my response and a reconstruction of the message I was about to deliver. It was as if I was connected to the divine Source inside of me on a whole new level. Suddenly, my higher self was helping me to be the person I always wanted to be. It was a collaboration between my Higher Power, my higher self, and the Universe - completely magical and completely inexplicable. However, if I had tried to understand meditation first, I would have never committed to the practice. I first had to take the action to gain the experience, then the understanding and the alignment of my thoughts followed.

One of my favorite sayings is *"You can't think your way into right action, but you can act your way into right thinking."*

Whenever I need to do something that I don't understand, I have found that the answer is to put my understanding aside and lean into the action. Once I take the action consistently, the understanding and positive feelings follow.

We live in a world where the power of intuition has been discounted and power has instead been relinquished to the mind and the intellect. This shift has convinced us that all the answers can be found in our brains, but that is simply untrue. I truly believe that it should no longer be a contest between the right brain and the left brain or the mind and the heart. It's about developing all of our abilities and harmonizing them to work together for our highest good.

Daily Practices & Action Plan

You now have the basic tools to start living a miraculous life!

You can now begin to write out your strategy so that this is not just some nice information you read about but a real plan to create lasting and sustainable changes in your life. From the ordinary to the miraculous, you must make this part of your daily living.

How do you do that? It's simple! Make a list of all the actions that you will take toward the manifestation of your miracle and write down your intentions with accompanying daily or weekly actions. However, you plan your schedule and your activities, make sure that you add the intention behind the action. Remember, it's not just the action that has power. It's the intention behind it that enhances or diminishes that power.

There are a few non-negotiable prerequisites for creating spiritually and emotionally fertile ground for these seeds to take root and grow. First, you create and commit to a morning routine. As human beings, we have inherited a brain from our stone-age ancestors that is particularly alert to the possibility of danger, so we are programmed to notice what's wrong with something before noticing anything else about it. Neuroscientists call this negativity bias. Maintaining a morning mediation/prayer practice is designed to overcome this negative bias and open our hearts to the blessings and miracles that our Higher Power is giving us each day.

Every spiritual tradition acknowledges that how we begin our day matters. I want you to pause for a moment and imagine this possibility. Why wake up each day with fear, stress, or panic about the enormity of the responsibilities that await us? What if we instead first open our eyes each morning to witness and recognize the Universe and our Higher Power's hand in the details of the day to come. If our very first expression is

161

gratitude - rather than seeing what's wrong or obsessing over how much work needs to get done - then we step onto the path of the miraculous and prepare ourselves for discovery, creativity, and peace.

It is much easier to create this practice than you might think. Upon awakening, the first thought you should have is, *thank you for another extraordinary day.* By stating that intention at the onset, you are already on your way to experiencing the day differently, to experiencing the miraculous.

Next, take a few moments for yourself. Find a quiet place to do a meditation (you can start with five minutes and expand from there). I highly recommend using a guided mediation app which can be downloaded on your phone or iPad. There are also many excellent morning meditations available on YouTube.

After your meditation, take another few moments to say a prayer. The secular definition of prayer is "An earnest request or wish." Start with giving thanks for what you already have and for what you know is on the way. Then ask for strength and guidance as you go about your day plus anything else you would like to add. Remember, this is not a religious practice and does not require religious beliefs. You are simply connecting with your higher self, your Higher Power, and the Universe. The only thing you need to know is that the sun comes up every day without your intervention. Try to connect to the power of nature and the Universe that is pulsating throughout the galaxies. But remember, don't try to understand it first. Take the action and the understanding will follow. When you hit challenges throughout the day, you can pause and ask your Higher Power to guide you.

Next is a journaling/writing practice. You will be amazed by how the power of journaling can unlock the secrets of your heart and mind and lead you directly toward your deepest desires. I highly recommend taking pen to paper, studies have shown that writing things out long hand versus typing them into our laptop or cell phone, allow us to tap into the area of our brain connected with learning and memories.

Write about your fears and insecurities as well as your dreams and desires. Make sure that you write in your journal about all the above at least weekly. Daily, you will also want to write down five things you are grateful for and five statements that affirm the person you want to be, your highest self. Write, for example, *"I am an award-winning chef!"* You may not yet be a chef, or if you are, you may not have won any awards yet, but if you affirm it and take action toward it, then it is only a matter of time before it becomes your reality.

How we end our day matters as much as how we begin it so, of course, you'll want to create a nighttime routine. There are so many studies on sleep hygiene and how preparing for a good night's sleep helps the quality of our sleep. I highly recommend spending 10 minutes each night before bed reading from a spiritual or inspirational book to wind down. You can search Amazon for some great authors in this genre such as Deepak Chopra and Marianne Williamson.

Lastly, I recommend sleep meditation. There are so many wonderful meditations available such as solfeggio and binaural beats. When I started listening to sleep mediation, I noticed that I fell asleep more quickly, slept more deeply, had fewer nightmares, and woke up more rested and peaceful. Sleep meditation is an opportunity for you to explore and expand your spiritual and creative side. Allow yourself to discover a whole new way to manifest and a whole new you along the way.

If you are having any doubts or fears, I suggest that you put them aside and fully give yourself to this experience. You cannot possibly know if it will work if you don't wholeheartedly do the work.

Judy Morris

You now have the basic tools to create a foundation to start living a miraculous life! I am so excited to see what you will discover about yourself and the Universe as you embark upon this spiritual healing journey.

My Gift to You

Now, as we have come to the end of this book, I want to leave you with a gift that the Universe has given me after over 20 years of doing this work:

I Am Not Broken Anymore

I am not broken anymore.
I am perfect whole and complete.
I know that and I feel it in every fiber of my being.
It is no longer a concept or something that I'm working toward.
It's no longer a destination that I hope to arrive to.
I am there.

I am no longer broken.
I love myself.
I take care of myself.
I don't look to others for my value, and I am no longer seeking to be saved.

I don't need you to need me to feel worthy of being here. I belong.
To myself and to my Higher Power who is not a person, place, or thing, he is the omnipotent, eternal benevolent Source energy that created me.
The master of the Universe designed me, he imbued me with special gifts, and talents.
He loves me, and is always with me, guiding me, comforting me, always and in all ways.

Judy Morris

I know that and knowing that is what strengthens me, stabilizes me, and guides me toward my highest truth - that I am not broken, abandoned, or alone.

I never really was.

What I was, was blind.
Blinded by my trauma.
Blinded by my pain.
Ignorant to the truth that I couldn't see because my vision had been obstructed by all the pain.

In healing the pain my sight returned.
As did my brilliance.

I am no longer drowning in darkness.
I can see the light because I am the light.
I am a miracle in the making and so are you.

Love,

Judy

Brittany Jones: Case Study

Brittany had always wanted to be successful. Her idea of success was to be financially independent, manifesting abundance in her business, and to be in a loving, affectionate, partnership that would ultimately lead to marriage and children.

She was a positive, happy-go-lucky person who was open to learning and growing. She had read lots of books on self-improvement and success, taken seminars, pursued several different businesses ideas, had dated and been in several long-term relationships, but found that she was unable to create the kind of results that she had always dreamed of. She would get to a certain level then plateau and burn out.

At 37 years old she had spent a decade falling in and out of love, with many different men and business ideas. She had been a bridesmaid countless times, and an aunt. She had witnessed her friends get engaged, then married, and start families. She watched them achieve their goals. And although she was happy for them, she was totally lost as to what the missing ingredient was that would turn the tide and launch her into her own dream life. She had run out of ideas, didn't know what to do next, and did not have a plan. She was starting to feel broken and kept asking herself: "what's wrong with me?"

Brittany had been doing all the "right" things, reading all the right books but she wasn't getting the results. She found herself in yet another dead-end relationship with a man of meager means, who was struggling in his business. He was chronically depressed and alcoholic. Brittany thought that maybe getting some coaching/support on how she might be able to empower him could help her, help him, and in turn allow them to create a beautiful life together.

She asked her best friend (who was happily married and running a thriving business) for suggestions on how to get the support she was looking for and her best friend gave her the best advice. She told her that she needed a coach and referred her to me.

When we sat down for our first meeting it became apparent to me that this lovely woman was very clear about the life she wanted. What she was clueless about what how to get there. And, on top of that, she had no idea how the decisions she was making and the actions she was taking were completely sabotaging her success.

Although she had read "all" of the books, taken all of the seminars, and "knew" lots of information, she hadn't learned how to implement all that information into her daily living. Knowing something and living something are as different as night and day. Just because you have a basic knowledge of something doesn't mean that you know how to implement it into your daily living and mindset.

During our first session I was able to help Brittany see the incongruency of her actions in relationship to her dreams and I helped her create a road map to get to where she wanted to go.

When I asked her if she was excited about this new journey she stated: *"Initially, I was scared. I was afraid if I really took all the actions and aligned my living with my goals that it wouldn't work out and I would discover that I was doomed to a life of mediocrity where I would never reach my potential or be fulfilled."*

However, her ticking biological clock coupled with the fatigue of chronic disappointment inspired her to draw a line in the sand and she declared that she would no longer allow insecurity and fear run the show. The "wait and see what happens" was a strategy for victims. She would never be the heroine of her life story hiding out on the sidelines. She threw her hat over the wall and hired me – GAME ON.

During our time together Brittany discovered the root of why she was continuing to manifest things she didn't want instead of what she did.

1. No clear understanding of how to implement the things she had learned into action and results

"I didn't date with discernment or intention; I didn't ask myself if the business lit me up and if its success structure was in alignment with my deepest desire. I was asking all the wrong questions. I was dating guys that were cute that I was attracted to — but that was as far as it went. I wasn't really vetting them to see if they were serious or would be husband/father material. I was jumping through hoops in business not asking myself if this activity brought me joy or if the activity was sustainable. I was giving of myself and not expecting a return on my investment of time and energy. It was a losing proposition."

2. No Life Plan

"I had no real idea how to attract my divine right partner or to discover the best business opportunity that would be a fit for my skills, interests, and abilities. I wanted to produce impressive results and I wanted to make an impact, but I had no idea how. I was just winging it." Discipline wasn't her strong point. So, she knew she needed support to clarify her goals, create a plan and then help keep her accountable along the way.

3. Not operating consistent with my value as a woman

"I lost sight of my value as a woman. Somewhere along the way, I began operating from insecurity so the crumbs that were being offered me romantically and professionally actually seemed appropriate. I had allowed my mistakes and failures define me. That coupled with unresolved childhood/family stuff, and I was living a life of some kind of penance sacrificing my dreams and settling for less."

After our first session Brittany got to the bottom of what was missing and got a plan in place. *"It was such a relief to discover that there is nothing wrong with me, the flaw has been in my lack of strategy, foggy vision, and lack of support."*

After just one session she had a clear blueprint toward her dreams.

A few months later she had not only gotten out of that dead-end relationship but left her dead-end job to pursue her dream career!

With the proper foundation in place, she was able to make the changes necessary to reach her goals.

Brittany not only created her dream career and the financial independence that she had always wanted, but she also manifested her divine right partner and got engaged!

"Having a crystal-clear road map to work from and the support of a coach who held my dreams as though they were her own, this allowed me to maintain my focus and align my actions toward my goals, helping me to finally create the life of my dreams."

Brittany didn't just get the man of her dreams, the Universe had something much bigger in store for her, she got a highly esteemed CEO who was also a multi-millionaire and has become a CEO herself, running a thriving 6-figure business while becoming the mother of a beautiful baby boy. She really does have it all and is living the life that she always wanted.

Michael Zaitsev: Case Study

Michael Zaitsev was beloved by his brother Anton who was extremely worried about him. Anton heard me speak at a workshop, approached me after the event, and quickly scheduled a call with me.

Anton was looking for support for his brother who he desperately wanted to help. Michael had once been a golf protégé who was headed for international fame, but his career was cut short by an injury that didn't allow him to play like he used to. He was so devastated by the loss of his career path and identity that he allowed his world to shrink smaller and smaller into mediocrity. Michael moved to Los Angeles and was helping his family with their real estate business, which he was not passionate about. He also worked part-time as a bartender and was entangled in a co-dependent relationship with a woman who wasn't his true love. He was unhappy and was abusing marijuana to numb his unhappiness as he binge watched Netflix on his days off. Anton adored his brother and felt powerless as he watched Michael become more and more disconnected, almost losing his spark completely.

When Anton asked me if I could help Michael, I told him that I could IF he wanted help. There is a myth that exists in our culture that if only the "right" person comes along they can "fix" the person who is hurting themselves. This is not true. The greatest coach, therapist, doctor, etc. in the world could be assigned to a person in pain and if that person doesn't understand that they need help and is resistant to the help then there is nothing that can be done. Each human being has free will and can exercise their agency in any way they choose, including to their own destruction. I made sure that Anton understood this clearly before I agreed to speak with Michael.

I was pleasantly surprised when I had my first contact with Michael because not only was he open, but he also actually really wanted help and just hadn't known how to go about getting any. He was excited to have someone to talk to who could help him navigate out of the inauthentic, unfulfilling life that he had manifested out of anger and resignation. He was hopeful for the first time in a long time that he would be able to re-imagine his goals and start utilizing his talents again.

Of course, Michael, like many of my other clients had no idea what his real problem was when we met. He knew he was unhappy; and he knew that he shouldn't be smoking so much weed and numbing out with movies, but he didn't know what else to do. He had truly come to believe that being a part-time bartender and associate to his family's real estate business was his life and that he should be happy and embrace it. He was not connected to the fact that he had given up on his dreams and himself and had settled for a life of convenience vs. a life of fulfillment. He didn't know that the best part of him had died when he was injured and because he didn't know he was dead walking around like a zombie he didn't know he could come back to life. We had to get to what the problem was, and we also had to get to what he really wanted in life, he had lost his sense of purpose.

Together, we were able to get to the source of the traumatic event (his injury) in the first session and not only were we able to get to the depth of the problem, but we were also able to create his roadmap out of his dead-end life toward the life of his dreams.

Michael said: *"I always knew I had an entrepreneur somewhere deep inside me, I just had no idea what how to develop it. I love my family and I want to support their business, but I just couldn't work in an industry that I dislike and have no passion for. It was not only robbing me of my energy and passion it was harming my relationships with my family because I started to resent them for making me do something that I didn't want to do. The whole dynamic was destructive and unsustainable. I'm so grateful to my brother for never giving up on me, for knowing me and seeing that I needed help and finding it for me. Judy's coaching, support, and guidance was indispensable in helping free myself from a life of misery and mediocrity to living the life of my dreams".*

During our sessions Michael was able to discover his passion for golf again and he realized that although he could no longer play the pro circuit, he could empower youth and coach them as they developed their talents, he could empower their success. That was the aha moment for him. Of course, once he had his aha moment his doubt and insecurity kicked in. We were able to work on his mindset and complete those things in the past that were still haunting him and robbing him of his freedom and self-expression. He finally realized that he really could be a coach! It was as if a door opened that lead him out of a dungeon and into the sunlight. He now had a path. Given he now had a path, a purpose, and a direction, he was able to quit smoking, because he didn't need to be numb anymore because he was excited about his life. And he was able to get honest about his relationship and finally had the courage to end it to focus on building his business. He was also able to help his family find a replacement for him so he could step away from the business without feeling guilty.

Michael not only began his own coaching business, but he also became one of the number one golf teachers in his geographic region working with schools and camps, offering private lessons as well. He took on other coaches and runs a 6-figure sports coaching business as well as an elite golf-program for youth. Shortly after solidifying his business success, he met his soul mate, and married her in their dream wedding on a gorgeous vineyard and they recently had their first child. She is an incredibly beautiful, intelligent, intuitive, feminine partner who is the perfect combination of softness and power. She is a successful businesswoman in her own right and heads up a prestigious marketing department for a major fortune 500 company. They truly are a power couple. Michael has never been happier, freer, or more empowered in his life.

Overall Summary: This client's problem was that he was chronically disappointed because he continued to fail to achieve his most precious goals. That constant failure to manifest his dreams left him unhappy/unfulfilled.

While some individuals may be in a dead-end job or relationship, struggling with addictions, or struggling in their sobriety, they have an idea of the kind of life that they want to have, but are unable to figure out how to get there. All their "best ideas" have failed, and they keep landing right back at square one. They may have tried therapy and possibly even benefited from it, connecting more deeply with their feelings, and identifying maladaptive coping mechanism, but it still fell short of helping them to achieve their dreams. Their dreams continue to seem out of reach.

They think that their circumstances are to blame and if they had better circumstances that they would be better. Although there is some truth to that, meaning if your highest calling is to be an art teacher and you are working as a waitress (circumstance) you will not be fulfilled. However, it is not just their circumstances that are a source of unhappiness, the root cause of their suffering is that they are disconnected from their highest selves. They are unhappy because they are living inauthentic lives of survival. They have created masks to hide behind, to survive, but what they keep attracting is a match for the mask, not a match for their deepest desires. Hence the result is that they continue to fall deeper and deeper into compromise and despair, further and further away from their passion, purpose, contribution, and fulfillment.

Judy Morris

Alicia Reed: Case Study

Alicia had grown up in a "Christian" household. She was taught to believe in God and did to an extent. However, this fragile belief became diminished as she experienced more and more abuse in her household at the hands of family members who were self-proclaimed "Christians." Alicia moved further and further away from any kind of faith and relied more and more on destructive habits such as alcohol and drug abuse ultimately becoming a full-blown addict/alcoholic.

Alicia's addiction escalated taking her to the depths of self-destruction and homelessness. She became more and more bitter and resentful. Was she not the victim of the violent and sexual abuse in her home? Had she not been robbed of a normal, loving supportive childhood. Was this not an excuse for her behavior?

Alicia thought that she had pulled herself out of the grips of addiction when she became pregnant with her first child. She stopped using and vowed to give her child a safe and supportive home unlike the one she grew up in.

Unfortunately, the stresses of being in an abusive relationship with a misogynist and under the thumb of a controlling father-in-law, caused Alicia to break under the pressure and she started using again. This led to her worst nightmare, being served divorce papers, and facing the possibility of losing custody of her child.

What happened to her dream of the picture-perfect family that she so desperately wanted to create?

Although she had a clear vision of what she wanted, Alicia was totally powerless of her maladaptive coping mechanism and had a significant amount of unresolved childhood trauma that was standing in the way of

177

her ability to be a stable parent. She checked herself into rehab but just couldn't stay sober. She kept asking herself why?

Alicia would go to 12-step meetings but didn't want to work the steps. She would get a sober mentor in name only but didn't want to risk trusting the person and really doing the work. She claimed to believe in God when the truth of the matter was, she was angry at God and didn't trust in a power greater than herself. She had been so busy relying on self, on drugs, and alcohol that she had lost her ability to believe in anything else. She would go to rehab, get to a certain level then fear would kick in and she would run.

At 28 years old Alicia had finally hit bottom and come to the realization that if she didn't let go of her "Lone Ranger" façade she wasn't only going to lose her child, she was going to overdoes and die. She didn't want to do that to her son. So, she finally went ALL IN.

Alicia had been referred to me by a counselor in a program that she was participating in.

When we sat down for our first meeting, she was cold and quiet. It became apparent to me that this was a woman who was paralyzed by fear. She knew that she wanted help, but she didn't know how to ask for it. When I confronted her about this she stood up and made a beeline for the door. I followed her to the door and said, *"I get it. I was afraid too. I am here to help. You are not alone; won't you please just give me a chance?"* Alicia burst into tears. Suddenly, the flood gates opened, and she let it all out. In that moment she became available to God's grace. During that first session I was able to help Alicia see the incongruency of her actions in relationship to her commitments and I helped her create a road map to get to where she wanted to go. I became her recovery coach and helped her let go of her past resentments about God and spiritual practices. She opened her heart to trusting in a Higher Power and really doing the work that was required to heal and change.

When I asked Alicia what was different this time she stated: *"Every time I worked with a counselor I felt like a number, I didn't know how desperately I needed to feel loved, to feel that someone was committed to me. Judy is that kind of person. When you sit down with her you can just feel that she loves you and wants to empower you more than anything else in the world, like that is her mission. It was weird. I never had an experience like that before. I just knew I could let my guard down and that I would be safe. This feeling grew and deepened over time. It was as if my Higher Power knew that I was finally ready to allow love into my life and that I finally had someone in my corner. There was something different about Judy that made me trust her."*

During our time together Alicia discovered the root of what had kept her stuck in a loop of self-destruction:

1. No clear understanding of how a lack of boundaries and self-respect lead to bad choices, abuse, poor self-esteem, and spiritual and emotional poverty

"I didn't know that being promiscuous was problematic nor did I realize how much it was eroding my self-esteem. I just thought I was a sexual person and that it wasn't a big deal to sleep around. I had no idea that being disconnected from my worth was attracting men that didn't value me. I also didn't realize that I was operating from insecurity and co-dependency. I had convinced myself that I just wanted to be in a relationship, what I didn't realize was that being chronically romantically involved with little time between partners or relationships didn't allow me the time to process any of the experiences I was having, nor did it allow to learn the lesson and move on from there. I was stuck in a repetitive loop of love and sex addiction fueled by loneliness, insecurity, and low self-

Judy Morris

esteem. I was looking for a man to love me, support me, and save me. I didn't know that I had to provide that for myself with my Higher Power holding my hand along the way."

2. No Life Plan

"I had been so busy surviving that I never learned how to dream or set goals. I had no knowledge of how to attract a healthy relationship or a financially rewarding job that would allow me to utilize my innate talents, skills, interests, and abilities. I wanted to be a sober, sane, mom, who was a productive member of society. I wanted to be of service, I just didn't know how. I realized that I needed loving support and guidance to clarify my goals, create a plan, and be supported along the way."

3. Operating backwards

"I thought that if I found someone to love me that then I could work on my healing. I had it all wrong. I first had to love myself and set boundaries to attract loving people into my life to help me along the way. I had allowed my trauma to define me, I had unresolved childhood/family stuff and I had been avoiding dealing with and I finally realized that if I didn't deal with it, it was going to deal with me. I was done allowing the sins of my family and the mistakes of my past to destroy my future."

"After working with Judy, I was finally able to muster the courage to face my trauma and do the work I had been avoiding. I learned how to take responsibility for my own healing and how to process and loosen the grip that the past had on me. I was able to take contrary action which used to terrify me, and I was finally able to develop a deep, rich spiritual life which included an intimate relationship with my Higher Power. I finally stopped judging myself so harshly and was able to find compassion for the Alicia who did what she had to, to survive. I discovered my wholeness and was able to heal so much. The flaw in my past attempts at recovery was

180

the lack of support. I had been trying to do it all on my own and that didn't work."

Alicia just celebrated 4 years sober, she is working in the field of recovery (which is her passion) and completing her education to be a therapist. She has a beautiful relationship with her son and a positive co-parenting relationship with her ex. She is in a healthy romantic relationship but above all has a healthy relationship with herself and a deep nourishing connection to her Higher Power.

With the loving support, guidance, and structure, she was able to take the necessary actions toward healing and maintain her sobriety.

Whether you believe it or not or understand it or not there is a divine intelligence at playing the Universe.

Case in point: The sun came up this morning and you had nothing to do with it. If you look around at the Universe, mother nature, the change in seasons, the turning of the tides, there is a divine intelligence behind all that is present in the natural world. Whether you call that God, mother nature, Source energy, it matters not. But to think that you can live in a world that is governed by immutable universal laws and not know them or how to work with them, is an illusion.

That would be the same as to say that I know nothing about an engine nor how do use the tools to repair an engine but I'm going to play mechanic and start taking things apart. It would be a disaster.

That is what happens to many of us in life. We don't understand anything about how to work with the energies at play and then we wonder why we have no power to manifest the lives we truly want.

You see, either you believe that the divine power of the Universe is a terrorist out to taunt you or you believe that it is omnipotent, benevolent, and supportive. Our relationship to Source gives us the quality of our experience of being alive and impacts our actions. If we understand that what we put out, comes back to us then we would not put out negativity because that is not what we want to attract back to ourselves. We should not seek to plant weeds in our own gardens.

If I believe that a terrorist is running the show, then I will live in a constant state of fear. I will feel all alone, and my anxiety will be high. Conversely, if I know that I was created with love and purpose and that my Higher Power created me to be happy, joyous, free, self-expressed and a contribution to the world then I will feel supported, loved, and inspired. This confidence will allow me to muster the courage necessary to cultivate my talents and abilities, living my best life.

In addition, another critical part to this is understanding that my parents are NOT my Higher Power. My biological parents were simply the vessels that carried me into this world. I come through them but not from them.

My true lineage is divine, and I am heir to all the most magnificent gifts that life has to offer IF I will only rightly relate myself to my Higher Power and the world.

This conversation is spiritual in nature philosophical in nature but not religious in nature. You are not required to have a religion, but I assert that you are required to have an empowered relationship with your creator to have an empowered experience in the world you live in.

Lawrence Thompson: Case Study

Lawrence signed up for an employment services group that I was teaching. He was middle aged, unemployed, and was dealing with some physical health challenges. He had served in the military when he was younger and was a typical Marine, confident, tough, and stubborn. Lawrence was clear about his goal – he wanted to get a job.

When we had our first one on one session, it became apparent that he was going to be difficult to work with. Lawrence wasn't coachable. He was filled with ideas about what he wanted to do and how he wanted to do it. He was convinced that he was a victim of circumstance and that if he could only get his way, everything would be fine.

He approached me more like a waitress then a career coach and was stuck in a loop of giving orders without realizing any results. He attended my group for several weeks and was becoming more and more irritable in his demeanor. I was getting ready to suggest that he stop attending and refer him elsewhere when I decided to try a different approach. I sat Lawrence down after class one day and asked him a question. *"Do you know that you are unavailable to be contributed to?"*

He didn't hear me the first time and tried to change the subject. I put my hand up, gesturing for him to stop, and repeated my question. He heard it the second time and started crying. This physical giant of a man, this Marine, looked deep into my eyes and cried. I told him that I knew that he had a drinking problem. He asked me how I knew, and I explained that he had disclosed his drug history during his intake and the information was in his case notes. He told me that he hadn't used drugs in a long time but that he couldn't stop drinking and given his other health issues, it was going to kill him. Given his behavior, I had a feeling that Lawrence had traded drugs for drink, and I was right. In fact, he was taken aback by my assertion given the timing that his doctor had recently admonished him about his drinking, and he was truly at a crossroads in his life. I shared with him about my battle with Alcoholism and sobriety.

I asked Lawrence if he had ever gone to AA meetings, and he had not. He used to go to cocaine anonymous meetings but never AA because he didn't think he had a drinking problem. We talked about his employment struggles and how his drinking was exacerbating his health issues which was in turn impeding his ability to work. I suggested that he focus on getting his physical health in order by getting his mental health in order and I asked him if he would go to a meeting with me. He agreed. We cried and prayed and hugged.

That was on a Friday, and I took Lawrence to his first meeting the following Tuesday. He heard the message and started attending meetings regularly. He not only got sober, but he stayed sober. His fiancé returned to him, his health improved, and he was able to get his dream job working for a major corporation in Arizona. Lawrence had always wanted to live in Arizona and the company he wanted to work for had just opened a brand-new office there. He was able to purchase a condo for himself and his now wife and is living the life he always dreamed of. As of the writing of this book Lawrence has been sober over 9.5 years.

During our time together Lawrence discovered the source behind his suffering:

1. No clear understanding of how his attitude and habits were negatively impacting his health, isolating him from community and blocking him from the abundance that the Universe would bestow upon him if he were open and available

"I really had no idea how bad my attitude had become. I was pushing people away without realizing it. Somewhere along the way I had become

so independent I had lost the ability to receive, or as Judy put it, I was unavailable to be contributed to. After we sat down and had that conversation about how my behavior had been impeding her from helping me achieve my goals, I was blown away by the realization that as cliché as it sounds, I had been my own worst enemy all along. The only thing standing in my way was me, and I just didn't know it"

2. Reacting and surviving vs. thriving and living

"I had sustained some pretty serious injuries during my time in the military. Those injuries lead to increased use of alcohol and pain pills to manage chronic pain, the pain and impairment from being on heavy much medication prevented me from seeking employment, I had learned to live on my tiny income. I was consuming cheap junk food and gaining weight which contributed to my declining health and sedentary lifestyle. On top of that my substance abuse made me more irritable and argumentative. My doctor kept warning me that I was going to be in a health crisis if I didn't stop drinking, I was on the verge of losing my relationship with my fiancé – my problems just keep snowballing and the worse I got the more my life seemed like Groundhog Day. Unbeknownst to myself, I had become a victim of my circumstances. I had allowed myself to become an observer of my life rather than a creator of it. I hadn't dealt with the emotional pain of past traumas and my unresolved emotional issues were exacerbating my physical health issues. I was stuck in survival mode and didn't even know it. I had forgotten how to dream, how to create goals and a vision for my life. I had no idea what the problem was so how could I know the solution. I was working with Judy with the intention of achieving my employment goals. Little did I know that I was going to achieve so much more. Just by having a non-bias outside professional look at my lack of results she was able to see what I couldn't see and help me pinpoint exactly what the barriers were to my success. Not only was I freed up to pursue and

achieve my employment goals, but I also improved every other aspect of my life, including achieving what had previously seemed impossible, real, sustainable sobriety."

3. Not operating with honor and integrity

"I lost sight of my value as a man. I stopped honoring myself, my health, my sobriety. Somewhere along the way, I began operating from resentment, unresolved pain, and anger. I had projected my unresolved issues onto those around me. I had allowed the injustices of my youth and the mistakes I made in reaction to it all to imbitter me. My anger and disappointment had come to define me. There was no chance of manifesting an inspiring future when I couldn't let go of the past."

"Working with Judy I not only got to the bottom of what was missing with regard to my career, but I got to see the big picture of what was impeding my success and was able to create structures and support to empower the fulfillment of my goals."

Appendix

If my book and work speak to you, I would love the opportunity to work with you further. I have a variety of offerings - online courses, group coaching, and one on one coaching.

However, if you need clinical intervention or simply have limited resources and want to start your healing journey today, I've included a list of resources below.

Addiction:

If you think you have a drinking problem and have thought about going to a meeting but have been too embarrassed to go in person, you can attend your first meeting virtually. Check out the website to find information and meetings in your area: www.aa.org

Not all treatment centers are created equal. If you're seeking treatment or would like to assist a loved one to get into treatment, contact an interventionist either online or in your area. They have a higher caliber of vetted professionals on their list than calling a toll-free number where a trained salesman (not a mental health professional) will sell you on their program based solely on whether or not they accept your insurance. It may cost a little more up front to work with an interventionist but the services they can provide to help you navigate the entire process will be well worth it in the long run. www.associationofinterventionspecialists.com

Kenneth M. Adams and Associates is a specialty practice treating sexual addiction and other intimacy-based disorders. Their staff is specifically trained and experienced to provide evidenced-based treatment in a safe, confidential, and respectful atmosphere. They offer a range of services to address the complex needs involved with these problems. www.sexualhealth-addiction.com

Career Services:

There are plenty of fine career coaches that you can find who offer various programs at reasonable costs. If you are unemployed or underemployed and cannot afford to purchase such service be advised that every state has basic job placement/vocational services and tuition assistance AT NO COST for veterans, and people with a disability. Depression and anxiety are qualifying disabilities. There is no cost or obligation to look into services. You can do an online search for the Department of Rehabilitation in your state to find out which services your state offers.

Domestic Violence Support:

Everyone deserves relationships free from domestic violence. Confidential support is available 24/7/365. www.thehotline.org or 1.800.799.SAFE(7233)

Family Services:

Al-Anon is a mutual support program for people whose lives have been affected by someone else's drinking. By sharing common experiences and applying the Al-Anon principles, families and friends of alcoholics can bring positive changes to their individual situations, whether or not the alcoholic admits the existence of a drinking problem or seeks help. www.al-anon.org

If you live in Illinois or the surrounding area, check out The Family Institute at Northwestern University: www.family-institute.org

The Center for Healthy Sex:

The Center for Healthy Sex is a certified team of dedicated professionals specializing in sex addiction treatment and sex therapy. Their sex therapists have over 22 years of experience treating issues such as sexual dysfunction, porn addiction, love addiction, and sex addiction in Los Angeles. They provide individual therapy, online coaching classes, couples therapy, group therapy, and workshops.
https://centerforhealthysex.com/www.centerforhealthysex.com

Therapists:

You can google sliding scale therapy in your city and state to find out what local resources are available. There are also online therapy solution available, including www.betterhelp.com

Judy Morris

Sources

Adams, Kenneth M.. *Silently Seduced: When Parents Make Their Children Partners. United States, Health Communications, Incorporated, 2011.*

APA Dictionary of Psychology, www.dictionary.apa.org/intergenerational-trauma. Accessed 11 July 2022.

Atlas, Galit. *Emotional Inheritance: A Therapist, Her Patients, and the Legacy of Trauma. United States, Little, Brown, 2022.*

Baz Luhrmann - Everybody's Free (To Wear Sunscreen) Lyrics | Lyrics.Com., www.lyrics.com/lyric/2968737/Baz+Luhrmann/Everybody's+Free+(To+Wear+Sunscreen). *Accessed 11 July 2022.*

Beattie, Melody. *Codependent No More: How to Stop Controlling Others and Start Caring for Yourself. United States, Hazelden Publishing, 2009.*

Buscaglia, Leo F.. *Living, Loving & Learning. United States, Fawcett Columbine, 1983.*

By GoodTherapy.org Staff. *"The Psychological Wounds of Domestic Violence." GoodTherapy.Org Therapy Blog, 17 Oct. 2014,* www.goodtherapy.org/blog/the-psychological-wounds-of-domestic-violence.

Day, Doris, et al. *Love Me or Leave Me* Warner Bros. Home Entertainment, 2020.

Dunaway-Seale, Jaime. "Bad Bosses Are Destroying Employee Happiness." *Real Estate Witch*, 14 Mar. 2022, *www.realestatewitch.com/employee-unhappiness-2022*.

Finkelstein, S. R., & Fishbach, A. (2012). Tell me what I did wrong: Experts seek and respond to negative feedback. *Journal of Consumer Research, 39(1)*, 22–38. *https://doi.org/10.1086/661934.*

Forleo, Marie. *Everything Is Figureoutable*. United Kingdom, Penguin Publishing Group, 2020.

Fox, Emmet. *The Sermon on the Mount: The Key to Success in Life*. N.p., Independently Published, 2019.

Gibran, Kahlil. *The Prophet*. Australia, Floating Press, 2009.

Gordon, Chad. "The Importance of Self-Awareness with Tasha Eurich." *Blanchard LeaderChat*, 1 Feb. 2019, *www.leaderchat.org/2019/02/01/the-importance-of-self-awareness-with-tasha-eurich*.

Harris, Nadine Burke. "How Childhood Trauma Affects Health across a Lifetime." *TED Talks*, 17 Feb. 2015, *www.ted.com/talks/nadine_burke_harris_how_childhood_trauma_affects_health_across_a_lifetime*.

*"Joseph M Carver, Ph.D. - Clinical Psychologist." www.drjoecarver.com,
www.drjoecarver.com. Accessed 11 July 2022.*

*Lamont, Penny. "SE 101." Somatic Experiencing® International, 29 Mar.
2022, www.traumahealing.org/se-101.*
*Llopis, Glenn. "6 Types of People Build Your Mental Toughness." Forbes,
15 Sept. 2012, www.forbes.com/sites/glennllopis/2012/07/23/6-
types-of-people-build-your-mental-toughness/?sh=42aa41fa561c.*

*McGraw, Dr. Phil. Self Matters: Creating Your Life from the Inside
Out. United Kingdom, Free Press, 2003.*

NCADV, www.ncadv.org. Accessed 11 July 2022.

NCJRS, www.ncjrs.gov/ovc_archives/ncvrw/2005/pg5f.html. Accessed 11
July 2022.

*Peterson, Jordan B.. 12 Rules for Life: An Antidote to Chaos. United
Kingdom, Random House Canada, 2018.*

*"Rewire Your Brain with Mindfulness." NeuroTrition, 30 Mar. 2016,
www.neurotrition.ca/blog/rewire-your-brain-mindfulness.*

*Rowling, J. K.. Very Good Lives: The Fringe Benefits of Failure and the
Importance of Imagination. United States, Little, Brown, 2015.*

*Van der Kolk, Bessel A.. The Body Keeps the Score: Brain, Mind, and Body
in the Healing of Trauma. United States, Penguin Publishing
Group, 2014.*

Judy Morris

Vidor, King, et al. The Wizard of Oz. Metro-Goldwyn-Mayer (MGM), 1939.

W., Bill. Alcoholics Anonymous: The Big Book. United States, Dover Publications, 2019.

W., Bill. Alcoholics Anonymous: The Story of how Many Thousands of Men and Women Have Recovered from Alcoholism. United States, Alcoholics Anonymous World Services, 1986.

W., Bill. Twelve Steps and Twelve Traditions Trade Edition. United Kingdom, Hazelden Publishing, 1953.

Ware, Bronnie. Top Five Regrets of the Dying: A Life Transformed by the Dearly Departing. United States, Hay House, 2019.

Williamson, Marianne. A Return to Love: Reflections on the Principles of A Course in Miracles. United States, HarperCollins, 2009.

Acknowledgements

Writing a book is a massive endeavor. An undertaking that cannot be done independently. In my experience, it requires a group of supportive individuals and professionals to empower the authors vision and ensure that he makes it across the finish line.

First and foremost, I want to thank my Higher Power for his unwavering faith in me, for providing an endless supply of love, inspiration, and guidance. My strength and power come from my creator. B'H.

I want to acknowledge my beloved Maxine Jarvis who was a dear friend and support in my life. Thank you for opening your home to me, and for showing me a love like none other I have ever experienced. Thank you for helping me get on my path and for being a cheerleader along the way. Although you're no longer on this earth, you are always with me as a guardian angel.

I want to acknowledge and appreciate my beloved Godfather, William MacDonald. He has been a surrogate father, best friend, and biggest supporter all my adult life. I could have never gotten this far without him. He has always believed in me in and my vision and has always stood by my side as I pursued my dreams and achieved my goals.

Thank you to my Imam, RC who has always seen through the façade of my ego, recognizing the real me and my untapped potential. Thank you for believing in me, pushing me, and guiding me towards the education that trained and developed me into the master coach that I am today.

Thank you to Dr. Bruce Derman, my very first therapist who became my mentor and dear friend. Thank you for holding my hand as I looked for the keys to unlock the doors of my psyche unearthing childhood trauma, dysfunctional relational patterns and a variety of other neuroses that were blocking me from living my best life. Thank you for your brilliance, patience, skill, and passion for what you do. Thank you for believing in me and being a most valued mentor and teacher. Your work is deeply imprinted in me, and I am eternally grateful for that.

Thank you to the brilliant leaders who trained and developed me: Gail Barnum, Elise Slifkin-Mcclure, Candace Shivers-Morgan, Jerry Burkhard, David Cunningham, David Botfeld, and Barry Pogorel. I am eternally indebted to you for your mastery and brilliance in training and developing me as a leader, teaching me the depth and power of integrity, the art and science of communication and the distinction coach.

I want to express my deepest gratitude to the women I have mentored over the years and to my clients. Thank you for your trust and your listening. Thank you for your courage to fight the fight. I have learned so much from you and have healed so much with you. I love each and every one of you (you know who you are) and am forever altered by our journey together.

Thank you to my treasured friend Kaitlyn Schoenleber. I cannot imagine trudging this road without you. You have been such an enormous blessing in my life. Your love, friendship and support have been so healing and empowering. Thank you for sitting with me for endless hours listening to all of my ideas. Thank you for being a sounding board and for your brilliant feedback and constant support. You are such a beautiful, bright light in this world I am so honored to have you by my side.

Thank you to my dear friends and beta readers Renee Kische and Ashley Morrison. Your friendship is priceless, and your support and feedback were deeply appreciated in this project.

Thank you to the community leaders who have inspired and supported me along my journey Harriet Bickle, Jeannie Marshall, Peter Greene, Robin Zeavin, Kay Getzoff, and Thomas Murphy. Thank you for being pillars of our community, for your integrity, unwavering love, and service. I am forever altered and blessed by your presence in my life. Thank you for leading the way.

Thank you to my treatment team: Dr. Michael Roth, Leanne Hunt, and Joanna Lawrence-Mills. Thank you for keeping me sane, helping me heal, and nurturing me. Your love, technical skill, healing prowess, and support are priceless to me. Thank you for keeping me well so I can continue to contribute to others.

A special shout out to my colleague and friend Frank Banos, without whom this book would not have been possible. Thank you for believing in me and supporting me to make this dream a reality.

Another special shout out to my beloved friend, Summer Swigart. We wear so many different hats in each other's lives. It is always an adventure. This book would not have been possible without you and your support. Thank you for believing in me and for pushing me out of my comfort zone and into the light. You're support of this book and my business have been instrumental in getting my message out to the masses in a much bigger way. Thank you for your trust and for your unwavering belief in me and the difference I make in the world.

I would also like to acknowledge my coaches and technical team. Thank you to Emma Hamlin of the Authors of Influence Academy for being a brilliant book coach and guiding me through this process from the quantum blueprint to my finished manuscript. Your program is such a gift to authors. Thank you to my personal coach Danielle Gray. Joining your program has been such a life-changing, transformational experience. Thank you for creating programs of impact that empower women to align to their highest selves to manifest their deepest desires. Your unwavering love and support have been instrumental in me fulfilling my dreams and taking my work out into the world in a much bigger way than I had before.

Judy Morris

Thank you to Elysia Skye for your presence in my life both professionally and personally, attending your content camp was life-changing and it led me to an incredible photographer Libby Danforth who I am so lucky to have worked with. She captured my message visually in a way that was so powerful. It was one of her photos of me that graces the cover of my book! And I can never thank you enough for introducing me to my beautiful, brilliant, and talented editor and publisher Megs Thompson.

Megs, you are so much more than an editor you are literally a book birthing midwife. Thank you for sitting with me for endless hours being a sounding board and helping me get clear about how to tell my story - making sure that my every word flowed. Thank you for designing my book cover and for sharing your many different talents with me. I am so deeply grateful for you and your magical gifts - you have been an incredible support, professional guide, and friend throughout this process.

Lastly, thank you to my brilliant and talented husband Scott Fresina of The Draw Studios Creative Arts Workshop. Thank you for being such a secure man who allows me all the space I need to continually transform myself, create impactful work for the world, and contribute to others. You are my biggest fan and cheerleader. Thank you for believing in me, for loving me and for always showing up and stepping up into the next best version of yourself to meet me and our marriage at its next stage of development. Your strength, humility, affection, and support fuel my soul and allow me to soar.

About the Author

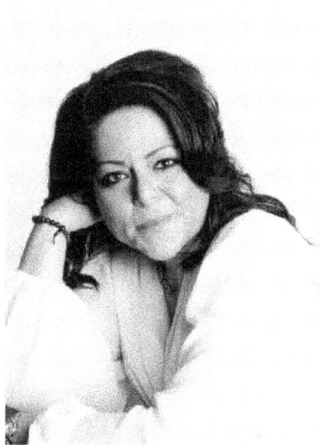

Judy Morris, a former Wall Street executive turned transformational coach/spiritual guide, public speaker, and author opted to leave the corporate world in 2010, after successfully recovering from her own major depressive disorder, childhood developmental trauma, and alcoholism. Dedicating her life and career to illuminating, advocating, and inspiring others to break free from the chains of addiction and challenges of mental health, Judy speaks on a variety of topics including recovery from substance abuse, codependency, and mental health issues.

Through her coaching business and speaking opportunities, Judy empowers hundreds of individuals on their journeys of healing and recovery, encouraging them to face their fears, connect with their higher selves, and begin the process of manifesting miraculous results in their own lives.

For more information about Judy or to explore her service offerings, visit her website at www.judymorriscoaching.com.